AF861498

Frank G McWilliams RN

INFECTIOUS DISEASES

4.50

INFECTIOUS DISEASES

BY 8 AUTHORS

EDITED BY J. JOSEPH MARR, M.D.

Assistant Professor of Medicine, Microbiology, and Pathology, Washington University School of Medicine; Director, Microbiology Laboratories, Barnes Hospital, St. Louis

LITTLE, BROWN AND COMPANY
BOSTON

Published November 1973

Copyright © 1973 by Little, Brown and Company (Inc.)

First Edition

All rights reserved. No part of this book may be reproduced in any form or by any electronic or mechanical means, including information storage and retrieval systems, without permission in writing from the publisher, except by a reviewer who may quote brief passages in a review.

Library of Congress catalog card No. 73-1424

ISBN 0-316-54665

Portions of the material in this book have appeared in condensed form in *Missouri Medicine*.

Printed in the United States of America

CONTRIBUTING AUTHORS

Unless otherwise noted, all authors are at Washington University School of Medicine and Barnes Hospital, St. Louis, Missouri.

MALCOLM T. FOSTER, JR., M.D.

Associate Professor and Vice-Chairman, Department of Medicine, University of Nebraska College of Medicine, Omaha

HALL E. HARRISON, M.D.

Internist and Cardiologist, Topeka, Kansas

OWEN S. KANTOR, M.D.

Assistant Professor of Medicine and Preventive Medicine

GEORGE S. KOBAYASHI, PH.D.

Associate Professor of Medicine and Assistant Professor of Microbiology; Associate Director, Microbiology Laboratories

J. JOSEPH MARR, M.D.

Assistant Professor of Medicine, Microbiology, and Pathology; Director, Microbiology Laboratories

GERALD MEDOFF, M.D.

Associate Professor of Medicine, Assistant Professor of Microbiology, and Chief, Division of Infectious Diseases

LEONARD N. NEWMARK, M.D.

Instructor of Clinical Medicine

PAUL M. SOUTHERN, JR., M.D.

Associate Professor of Pathology and Medicine, The University of Texas Southwestern Medical School at Dallas; Director of Clinical Microbiology, Parkland Memorial Hospital, Dallas

PREFACE

INFECTIOUS DISEASES are among the most common problems that present themselves to the physician. Many of them can be treated only symptomatically, while others are amenable to specific therapy. Another group of illnesses has emerged which is itself a reflection of progress made in other disciplines, this new group being the opportunistic infections. It is the contention of those of us who deal principally with infectious diseases that in treating all of these groups there is a tendency to bring about immediate symptomatic relief to the patient rather than to delve into the nature of the infectious process. This is said not to deprecate attempts at therapy but to emphasize that immediate treatment often obscures the actual underlying process and renders definitive action more difficult. The presence of an infection in an otherwise apparently healthy individual frequently is a warning that host defense mechanisms have been compromised. It is the underlying disorder that must be sought and, if possible, corrected. In the ensuing chapters we have endeavored to stress this approach by giving emphasis to pathophysiology and to methods of arriving at a diagnosis. Comments regarding therapy, although of obvious value, have been given less importance.

We would like to thank all those who have helped to bring our efforts to fruition. They include the many individuals who were kind enough to review and criticize the various chapters as well as those who assisted in the mechanics of preparing the manuscript, in particular, Mrs. Mary Johnson, who faithfully converted twelve chapters of illegible manuscript into final copy.

My contributions to this book were supported in part by a grant from the National Science Foundation (GB-36052).

J. J. M.

CONTENTS

CONTRIBUTING AUTHORS v

PREFACE vii

1 / GENERAL CONSIDERATIONS
J. Joseph Marr 1

2 / THERAPEUTIC ALTERNATIVES TO PENICILLIN
J. Joseph Marr 7

3 / MODIFICATION OF ANTIBIOTIC REGIMENS IN RENAL FAILURE
J. Joseph Marr 17

4 / PULMONARY INFECTIONS
Paul M. Southern, Jr. 31

5 / BACTERIAL MENINGITIS
J. Joseph Marr 53

6 / URINARY TRACT INFECTIONS
J. Joseph Marr 73

7 / GRAM-NEGATIVE SEPTICEMIA
Malcolm T. Foster, Jr., and Owen S. Kantor 87

8 / BACTERIAL ENDOCARDITIS
Malcolm T. Foster, Jr., and Hall E. Harrison 97

9 / MANAGEMENT OF TUBERCULOSIS
IN THE COMMUNITY HOSPITAL
J. Joseph Marr 113

10 / OPPORTUNISTIC INFECTIONS
Gerald Medoff and George S. Kobayashi 129

11 / STREPTOCOCCAL DISEASE
Leonard N. Newmark 143

12 / VENEREAL DISEASE
J. Joseph Marr 155

INDEX 173

INFECTIOUS DISEASES

1 / GENERAL CONSIDERATIONS

J. Joseph Marr

THE STUDY of infectious diseases impinges upon the general field of internal medicine in many areas, and, in succeeding chapters, an attempt has been made to demonstrate the relationship between the interests of the specialist and the needs of the generalist. The commonly accepted principles of therapeutics and patient management have been assumed in discussing the disease entities, and only those variations in therapy or clinical practice have been emphasized which are of particular importance in the management of a particular illness. In this introductory statement a few guidelines are given which may be of assistance in ordering one's approach to a patient with an infectious disease. Although it is recognized that there is little that is absolute in biology, these suggestions are presented somewhat dogmatically for the sake of emphasis.

Perhaps the cardinal concept in the use of antimicrobial agents is that no drug, whether bacteriostatic or bactericidal, will be curative in and of itself. Therapy should be chosen after consideration of the nature of the infecting organism, its rate of multiplication, and the status of the host's defense mechanisms. The physician's evaluation of these considerations, through his initial clinical and laboratory assessment of the patient, is of major importance in the subsequent management of an infectious disease. When possible, therapy should be initiated only after the identification of the etiologic agent; this is frequently based primarily on clinical information (site and duration of infection, underlying illnesses, previous therapy, and so on), but confirmatory laboratory data should always be sought. The major immediate laboratory aid is the gram stain. Common errors in the use of this method are overdecolorizing and misinterpretation of precipitated stain as showing gram-positive cocci. Placing a small amount of gingival scrapings on the slide along with the material in question is a good precaution. The mouth contains many gram-positive and gram-negative organisms, and the finding of both in this control section of the slide assures the physician that it is properly stained.

The gram stain only provides a general indication as to an organism's identity, and adequate methods of culturing must be used as well. Techniques peculiar to particular disease processes will be discussed in later sections; however, a few general rules may be stated.

1. When bacteremia exists or can be anticipated by a recurring fever pattern, cultures are most productive when taken just prior to or during a chill.
2. Pour plates of blood cultures sometimes will provide a more rapid means of identification of the offending pathogen and will give an indication of the numbers of bacteria present. Contaminating organisms are discovered easily with this technique, whereas they may cause confusion if permitted to grow freely in a bottle of liquid medium. Use of pour plates also provides the physician with a means of following the results of therapy in terms of a decreasing number of organisms per milliliter of blood when a clinical response is not yet evident.
3. Saliva should not be cultured. If sputum cannot be coughed up, then transtracheal aspiration should be done to obtain an uncontaminated specimen (see Chapter 4).
4. Body fluids should be cultured immediately, since a delay will permit fastidious organisms to die and contaminating organisms to proliferate.

Frequently it is necessary to begin treatment before the results of cultures are obtained, so a knowledge of the most probable infecting organism is requisite. A list of some of the etiologic agents of the more common adult infections is presented in Table 1-1. The table serves only as a guide, since the clinical evaluation of the patient will modify the possibilities in any given individual.

The importance of sensitivity testing of organisms known for their innate ability to develop resistance to antibiotics cannot be overemphasized. Routine sensitivity determinations of organisms known

TABLE 1-1 / Microorganisms Commonly Isolated from Acute Adult Infections

SKIN AND SUBCUTANEOUS TISSUES	**LUNGS**
Staphylococcus aureus	*D. pneumoniae*
Streptococcus pyogenes (group A)	*Mycoplasma pneumoniae*
Dermatophytes and *Candida albicans*	Respiratory viruses
	Haemophilus influenzae
DECUBITUS ULCERS	**URINARY TRACT**
S. aureus	*Neisseria gonorrhoeae* (urethra)
Escherichia coli	*E. coli*
	Other gram-negative organisms
PARANASAL SINUSES	*S. aureus* (after surgery)
Diplococcus pneumoniae	*Strep. faecalis*
Strep. pyogenes (group A)	**MENINGES**
S. aureus	*D. pneumoniae*
EAR	*N. meningitidis*
EXTERNAL	*S. aureus* (after neurosurgery)
S. aureus	Gram-negative organisms (particular instances)
Strep. pyogenes (group A)	**BONES (OSTEOMYELITIS)**
D. pneumoniae	*S. aureus*
MIDDLE	*Salmonella* species
Viruses	**JOINTS**
D. pneumoniae	*S. aureus*
S. aureus	*Strep. pyogenes*
	N. gonorrhoeae

to be susceptible to a given antibiotic, e.g., pneumococcus and group A streptococci, need not be carried out. However, the use of antibiotic discs, the most common laboratory method, may not give information about the clinical efficacy of the drug; the discs serve merely as a guide in the choice of an appropriate agent. In serious infections, such as subacute bacterial endocarditis, serial dilutions of the patient's serum should be assayed to determine if there is sufficient antibiotic present to produce a bactericidal effect in vivo. Infection is usually controlled when a dilution of serum of 1:8 or higher demonstrates a bactericidal effect on a standard test inoculum. Organisms in a rapid phase of growth will take up an antimicrobial agent and be inhibited by it more rapidly than organisms that are metabolizing slowly. The clinical corollary to this is that indolent infections such as subacute bacterial endocarditis will require long periods of chemotherapy. Failures in treatment of these types of infections are usually not due to inability to attain a sufficient concentration of antibiotic in the serum but to an early cessation of therapy.

The physiologic status of the patient is important in the choice of therapy, its route of administration, the rapidity with which treatment is initiated, and the possibilities of drug toxicity due to associated disease. For example, a patient with an immunologic deficiency or one infected with an organism capable of rapid growth (streptococcal cellulitis) or virulent either by virtue of its locus of infection (meningitis) or the toxic substances it produces (gas gangrene) should be treated with a bactericidal drug. A person less ill might be treated with a bacteriostatic agent.

Bactericidal agents complex with or prevent the formation of molecules that are not readily replaceable by the cell: DNA (nuclear or cytoplasmic), RNA, or cell membrane, or they prevent cell wall synthesis or inhibit formation of an enzyme crucial to the synthesis of one of the above (e.g., rifampicin inhibits bacterial RNA polymerase). Bacteriostatic agents structurally resemble physiologic compounds and act as competitive inhibitors in a metabolic sequence. By definition, competitive inhibitors can be replaced by the substances with which they compete; thus, the concentration of these antimicrobial agents and their duration of administration may become important. There is obviously much overlap between the two classes of drugs; moreover, the conditions under which the drug acts may convert a bactericidal agent into one which is *effectively* bacteriostatic; penicillin, the classic example of a bactericidal agent, may become bacteriostatic when the organisms are in the hyperosmolar environment of the renal medulla.

As a rule, bactericidal agents reinforce one another, whereas the combination of a bactericidal and bacteriostatic agent usually is antagonistic (e.g., penicillin and chloramphenicol). The weaker bacteriostatic agent will slow the growth of the organisms and thus render them more resistant to the bactericidal drug. This has been demonstrated experimentally and appears to be true clinically as well. A listing of the drugs in both groups is given in Table 1-2.

In serious infections and in any situation in which parenteral absorption of the drug may be altered, antimicrobial agents should be given intravenously. Intramuscular or oral therapy may be used in less demanding circumstances, but oral therapy is preferred when possible. Before using the oral route one should be certain that uniform absorption of the drug can occur; that the patient is taking nothing that might interfere with the absorption of the drug; and

TABLE 1-2 / Known Mechanisms of Action of Antimicrobial Agents

Agent	Mechanism of Action
BACTERICIDAL	
Penicillins	Inhibition of cell wall synthesis
Cephalosporins	Inhibition of cell wall synthesis
Vancomycin	Inhibition of cell wall synthesis
Bacitracin	Inhibition of cell wall synthesis
Aminoglycosides	Inhibition of protein synthesis
Polymyxins	Detergent action on cell membrane
BACTERIOSTATIC	
Chloramphenicol	Inhibition of protein synthesis
Erythromycin	Inhibition of protein synthesis
Lincomycin	Inhibition of protein synthesis
Tetracyclines	Inhibition of protein synthesis
Nalidixic Acid	Inhibition of DNA synthesis
Rifampicin	Inhibits bacterial RNA polymerase
Sulfonamides	Competes with para-aminobenzoic acid
Nitrofurantoin	Unknown

that blood levels of the orally administered antibiotic can be obtained that are equivalent to those secured by the parenteral route. The last criterion incorporates the others and, if it can be met, then oral therapy should be adequate.

The rapidity with which therapy is instituted depends entirely upon the clinical situation. Many times the question may be asked, "Is the risk of withholding therapy greater than that involved in starting it?" If answered affirmatively, treatment should be instituted; if not, there may be much to gain by waiting until a definitive diagnosis is made. When a decision is made to treat immediately, therapy should be as complete as possible; partial therapy or temporizing is not indicated.

Associated diseases may influence therapeutic decisions. Bactericidal agents should be used in patients with impaired host defense mechanisms (for example, patients with hematologic malignancies, those receiving corticosteroids or antimetabolites, patients with malnutrition or increased age). Factors influencing the dosage of an antibiotic frequently resolve themselves into the presence of associated liver or renal disease and, in these cases, the pharmacology of the drug assumes a greater importance. For example, a biliary tract infection is best treated by an agent which is excreted by the liver; in the presence of cirrhosis, drugs must be chosen that are not metabolized or excreted primarily by the liver. The most difficult management problem is the patient with renal insufficiency. The doses of antibiotics used in these individuals are usually reduced in parallel with the creatinine clearance, and hemodialysis or peritoneal dialysis may further alter the regimen. The dosage modifications necessary for treatment of a patient with renal disease are described in Chapter 3.

When a patient does not respond to the appropriate agent, the reasons for selecting the current therapy must be reconsidered. If no obvious changes are indicated, then the following questions should be asked.

1. Is a previously unsuspected abscess present?
2. Is the fever due to a drug reaction?
3. Has the organism developed resistance by enzyme induction, by R factor transmission, or by becoming cell-wall deficient?
4. Is the antibiotic penetrating the body space in which the infection is located?
5. Is a superinfection present?
6. Is the isolated organism really the etiologic agent?

Although the foregoing comments have been somewhat arbitrary, accumulated experience has shown that they encompass most of the problems associated with the management of an infectious process. Many of the topics which have been mentioned only in passing will be considered in detail in the following chapters.

2 / THERAPEUTIC ALTERNATIVES TO PENICILLIN

J. Joseph Marr

THE PHYSICIAN has at his disposal a variety of antimicrobial agents useful in the treatment of infections caused by gram-positive organisms. In most of these infections penicillin G is the drug of choice; however, there are many instances in which penicillin cannot be used because of resistance on the part of the organism or because of allergy on the part of the patient. In the former situation a semisynthetic penicillin will frequently be of value; in the latter circumstance the macrolide antibiotics, vancomycin, or lincomycin and its derivatives might be used. Because of the number of agents and their variations in mechanisms of action, side effects, and dosage, they will be presented as clinically related groups of drugs and discussed in that manner.

THE SEMISYNTHETIC PENICILLINS

Penicillin G. This agent has been in use clinically for the past 30 years, and it remains the most effective and least toxic of all available antimicrobial agents. If a choice exists between penicillin and an alternate drug, the former should always be used. The rapid renal excretion of penicillin is a disadvantage, although in urinary tract infections this property may be used to convert high serum levels to even higher urine concentrations. The development of the semisynthetic penicillins has extended the spectrum of these agents to include many gram-negative organisms not previously susceptible to concentrations which could be obtained clinically. The various preparations of the penicillins are prepared by chemical or biological modification of the 6-aminopenicillanic acid nucleus. Although there are many possible variations on this molecule, only the most widely used will be described.

The first preparation to exhibit activity against gram-negative organisms was ampicillin. It has the advantage of being excreted in the bile in high concentrations and is subject to enterohepatic recirculation. It is well absorbed when given orally, and its ultimate excretion is through the kidney. These properties make it a useful agent in both urinary tract and biliary tract infections. This drug is susceptible to staphylococcal penicillinase and is therefore not indicated when infection by these organisms is under consideration. It is, however, effective against *Haemophilus influenzae, Proteus mirabilis, Salmonella* and *Shigella* species, and most *Escherichia coli.* It generally is not used against gram-positive organisms since penicillin G and penicillin V are cheaper and more effective.

Carbenicillin. This drug has been recently released for clinical use. It has an antibacterial spectrum similar to that described for ampicillin and, like ampicillin, is susceptible to penicillinase. It has the decided advantage of being effective against *Pseudomonas aeruginosa* and *Proteus* species resistant to ampicillin. It is not efficacious against *Klebsiella* and is less effective against gram-positive cocci than other penicillins. The major use of carbenicillin is in the treatment of urinary tract infections, and this will be discussed in more detail in Chapter 6.

Methicillin. The prototype of the penicillinase-resistant penicillins, methicillin was first used clinically to halt the epidemic spread of virulent penicillinase-producing staphylococci in hospitals in 1959 [1–3]. Methicillin still remains an excellent agent against the penicillinase-forming staphylococcus because of its high stability to the enzyme [4]. Despite this, its activity is relatively low, only about 1% that of penicillin G. Moreover, the drug brings about induction of the enzyme and has only a fraction of the activity of penicillin G against nonpenicillinase-producing staphylococci and other gram-positive cocci. Therefore, methicillin is of value principally against penicillinase-producing staphylococci, and infection by these organisms is the sole indication for its use. The practice of giving methicillin along with penicillin G in infections due to gram-positive cocci cannot be recommended. The former provides only a small additive effect and may result in the induction of a penicillinase in organisms which have only small amounts of the enzyme to begin with. Although this finding remains primarily a laboratory phenomenon, the author believes that if the clinical situation indicates that infection by one of several gram-positive cocci is a possibility (e.g., orbital cellulitis) and that resistant staphylococci may be among the potential invaders, then one of the isoxazolyl penicillins or nafcillin should be used (see following section). As with any of the penicillinase-resistant drugs, if subsequent testing indicates that the organism does not produce penicillinase, then administration of the drug should be discontinued and penicillin G substituted. This is becoming of increasing importance since resistance to methicillin has appeared among some staphylococci in this country.

Allergic reactions to methicillin occur with a frequency similar to that of reactions to penicillin G, and cross-sensitivity to the latter should be anticipated. Idiosyncratic reactions are unusual, but a few cases of agranulocytosis have been reported [5]. Agranulocytosis due to methicillin is not a contraindication to the use of the other semi-synthetic penicillins. Nephritis occurs occasionally but is not common.

The Isoxazolyl Penicillins. These agents (oxacillin, cloxacillin, dicloxacillin) and nafcillin have been a significant addition to the therapeutic armamentarium. However, these drugs should be withheld unless one is treating an infection caused by a penicillinase-producing staphylococcus or when the probability exists that the infecting organism will produce this enzyme.

The common feature of this group of agents is the presence of a bulky, electron-attracting substituent on the side chain of the 6-aminopenicillanic acid nucleus. These additions decrease the susceptibility of the penicillin to hydrolysis by penicillinase, presumably through steric hindrance at the site of attachment to the enzyme. This group of drugs is acid-stable and thereby enjoys the advantage of oral administration. Despite numerous claims, no preparation appears to have clear advantages over another against penicillin-resistant staphylococci. The theoretical advantage of these agents over methicillin lies in their effectiveness against gram-positive organisms other than staphylococci. They are perhaps ten to twenty times more active than methicillin, although they are somewhat more toxic and less stable to the action of penicillinase.

Oxacillin should be given on an empty stomach, since its absorption is very unpredictable otherwise. When taken properly, about 60% is absorbed, and peak serum levels are attained in one hour. Intramuscular injection provides serum levels twice those obtained by the oral route with a great deal more certainty. This drug is excreted in the bile as well as in the urine, as are the rest of the semisynthetic penicillins. Since enteric absorption is somewhat erratic, oxacillin should always be used parenterally when serious infection is to be treated. Transaminase elevations and cholestatic jaundice have been reported.

Cloxacillin, the chlorphenyl analogue of oxacillin, is essentially identical to the parent compound in its therapeutic dimensions. It does offer the advantage of uniform absorption from the intestine with higher peak serum levels and a more sustained action than oxacillin. Therefore, it is to be preferred when oral therapy is used.

Nafcillin is about equivalent to cloxacillin in its therapeutic efficacy. Some workers [6] believe that nafcillin is somewhat superior to the other semisynthetic penicillins in the treatment of infection caused by gram-positive cocci other than the penicillinase-producing staphylococci. However, oral absorption is erratic, and the parenteral route is preferred.

The use of the semisynthetic agents should be restricted to infections caused by penicillinase-producing staphylococci or in instances when infection with these organisms is a possibility but infection by other gram-positive cocci must also be considered. In the latter case, one of the isoxazolyl penicillins or nafcillin should be used in preference to methicillin. Methicillin should only be used after isolation of the organism and sensitivity testing have indicated that it is a penicillinase-producing staphylococcus sensitive to the drug. Use of this drug against other gram-positive cocci may give poorer therapeutic results.

CEPHALOSPORINS

Agents belonging to this group are derivatives of 7-aminocephalosporanic acid and are quite comparable to the extended spectrum penicillins. They are not broad-spectrum antibiotics and should not be used as such. Their superiority to the penicillins lies in the fact that they are resistant to hydrolysis by penicillinases, except when the enzymes are present in high concentrations, and that they may be used in individuals known to be allergic to penicillin. Since these drugs were first introduced in 1964, a considerable amount of clinical experience has accumulated to document their effectiveness in the treatment of a variety of infectious processes.

The antigen which produces anaphylactic reactions to penicillin is associated with the opening of the beta-lactam ring of the 6-aminopenicillanic acid nucleus. However, the hydrolysis of this moiety in the cephalosporins results in fragmentation of the molecule. Thus, cross-sensitivity does not occur to a great extent. There is, nevertheless, about a 10 to 20% incidence of cross-reactivity, so cephalosporins cannot be considered a totally safe substitute for penicillin.

These agents have a definite place in the treatment of infection caused by penicillinase-producing staphylococci, *Klebsiella* infections, and in treating persons known to be allergic to penicillin. The antistaphylococcal activity of the cephalosporins is comparable to that obtained with the penicillinase-resistant penicillins [7]. They probably should not be considered the drugs of choice for infections other than the above. For most infections, penicillin and ampicillin are more effective, less expensive, and remain the drugs of choice.

Cephalothin. This drug is not absorbed orally; it must be given parenterally, 4 to 12 gm. per day in divided doses. For mild infections 1 gm. every 4 to 6 hours is adequate. Larger quantities are required for infections due to gram-negative organisms such as species of *Klebsiella. Pseudomonas* organisms are generally resistant to cephalosporins. For intravenous infusion, the drug is dissolved in about 40 ml. of 5% dextrose or isotonic saline and given over a 30-minute period. Ninety-five percent of the drug is excreted in the urine in about 6 hours, and it is distributed in all body fluids, although it does not cross normal meninges. Serum concentrations are enhanced by administering probenecid.

Cephaloridine. The pharmacologic and therapeutic properties of this drug are similar to those of cephalothin. The drug is excreted by the kidney and has been shown to cause renal tubular damage which appears to be cumulative and related to the dose. It is apparently secreted by tubular transport mechanisms which are not required for cephalothin excretion. Quantities of more than 4 gm. per day should be avoided.

Cephalexin. The development of this agent represents an attempt to combine the side chain of ampicillin with the nucleus of a cephalosporin in order to gain the advantages of both drugs. It is a bactericidal antibiotic which is well absorbed following oral administration, is not significantly bound to serum protein, and is excreted unaltered by the kidneys. Metabolic degradation is not extensive, and nearly all of the antibiotic is recovered in the urine in active form. After oral administration peak serum levels occur at 1 hour and persist for 4 to 6 hours. These serum concentrations are comparable to those obtained with intramuscular injections of cephaloridine and cephalothin [8, 9]. Cephalexin is useful in the treatment of many acute infections caused by gram-positive organisms, although it is not superior to an oral penicillin and its cost is substantially greater. Chronic infections, for example bronchitis and pyelonephritis, do not respond as well. It is useful in the treatment of urinary tract infections in outpatients caused by organisms which are resistant to other antibiotics.

Toxic reactions to cephalothins include the development of a positive Coomb's test, rarely with hemolytic anemia (this is a dose-dependent phenomenon). Reversible renal tubular necrosis has been described with cephaloridine, usually in doses in excess of 4 gm. a day. Pain and sterile abscesses at injection sites have been described with cephalothin; cephaloridine appears to be much less irritating in this regard.

MACROLIDE ANTIBIOTICS AND LINCOMYCIN DERIVATIVES

These agents are quite distinct chemically, although similar in their pharmacologic and therapeutic properties. All of these agents are active against gram-positive cocci, and their principal usage should be restricted to treatment of infections caused by these organisms. They have been generally considered to be bacteriostatic by virtue of their action in inhibiting protein synthesis, although in higher concentrations they are bactericidal [10]. Of the macrolide antibiotics, erythromycin has been more extensively studied and more widely used than has either oleandomycin or triacetyloleandomycin. This is due to the earlier appearance of erythromycin as well as its demonstrable superiority over the other macrolides in the treatment of infections caused by gram-positive bacteria.

Resistance to erythromycin is due to enzyme induction, and extends to oleandomycin and to lincomycin. Both the macrolides and lincomycin derivatives are widely distributed in the body and give high tissue concentration; however, they do not cross normal or even inflamed meninges to any great extent. Excretion is about 20% in the urine with the remainder in the bile. Side effects of erythromycin are uncommon and relatively minor: abdominal pain, nausea, vomiting, and diarrhea are seen most frequently and occur in approximately 2% of those taking the drug. Gastroenteritis is seen with all of the macrolides and lincomycin but is perhaps less prevalent with the latter. Although the macrolides are effective against some neisseriae, listeriae, and rickettsiae, lincomycin is not.

Erythromycin. Of about thirty-five known macrolides, only erythromycin and oleandomycin are used to any great extent. Only the former will be described, since it is less toxic and more effective on a weight basis. It is seldom the agent of choice in bacterial infections unless the infecting organism is resistant to penicillin or the patient is allergic to penicillin and the infection is not severe enough to require parenteral therapy. If an oral agent is to be used in the treatment of a mild gram-positive infection, then erythromycin might be preferred to penicillin since it appears to cause less gastrointestinal irritation.

Inasmuch as high tissue concentrations may be achieved with low toxicity, erythromycin is also a good agent for therapy of infections caused by wall-deficient organisms. This is true for gram-negative wall-deficient variants as well, since an intact cell wall appears to be responsible for the resistance of these organisms to the macrolides.

Two oral preparations of erythromycin are available: propionyl erythromycin lauryl sulfate (erythromycin estolate) and erythromycin stearate. Erythromycin estolate produces higher and more reliable blood levels than the stearate. However, the estolate preparations have been associated with a reversible cholestatic hepatitis. When this occurs, it is usually in patients who have received the drug for more than 10 to 14 days [11, 12]. This form of hepatitis may actually mimic an acute abdominal crisis. The syndrome will usually resolve on withdrawal of the drug. The consensus at this time is that the hepatitis represents an idiosyncratic reaction to the lauryl sulfate moiety and is not a dose-related toxic effect. During the past seven years there have been only about 200 cases reported. The same reaction has followed the use of oleandomycin esters. No toxic reactions of significance have been associated with the erythromycin base. The small possibility of a reversible cholestatic hepatitis is probably outweighed by the greater reliability of absorption of erythromycin estolate.

Although the use of erythromycin is declining due to the availability of penicillin G and synthetic penicillins, it appears to retain significant value in the therapy of chronic bronchitis and pneumonia caused by *Mycoplasma pneumoniae.* This organism is sensitive to both erythromycin (0.125 μg. per milliliter) and the tetracyclines (1.5 μg. per milliliter). A study by Rasch and Mogabgab [13] in which 105 cases of atypical pneumonia were treated alternately with erythromycin and tetracycline indicated that radiographic improvement occurred somewhat more rapidly with erythromycin than with tetracycline. No other significant differences in the clinical course were noted.

Lincomycin. This agent is an antibiotic with a structural configuration different from that of other antimicrobial agents. Like the macrolides, it inhibits bacterial growth by interfering with protein synthesis. Its antimicrobial spectrum is relatively narrow, resembling that of erythromycin, and it is active in a concentration of about 2 to 5 μg. per milliliter or less. Like erythromycin, lincomycin is bacteriostatic; however, bactericidal levels may be obtained at concentrations about thirty times those required to produce bacteriostasis. About 20 to 35% of an oral dose of lincomycin is absorbed from the gastrointestinal tract in the fasting state. The administration of 500 mg. by this route produces an average peak plasma value of about 0.5 to 2 μg.

per milliliter. Antibiotic activity reaches its height at 2 to 4 hours and is still present at 12 hours. Oral administration following meals reduces serum levels by about 50% [14]. Lincomycin is diluted in the body through a volume approaching the total weight. Although it does not penetrate the blood–brain barrier to any significant degree in patients with normal meninges, in the presence of meningitis cerebrospinal fluid concentrations may be as much as 40% of plasma levels.

In essence, the drug is pharmacologically and therapeutically the same as erythromycin. It offers no particular advantages with the possible exception that it may produce higher concentrations in bone and therefore be of use in treating osteomyelitis. Despite the fact that there has been a considerable investigation of lincomycin with regard to its ability to penetrate bone, the results remain somewhat conflicting. It is clear that this antibiotic will penetrate bone perhaps to a greater extent than even penicillin, but it is not yet certain that the drug is any more effective at the site of the osteomyelitis than are lower concentrations of penicillin.

Clindamycin. The 7-chloro analogue of lincomycin, clindamycin has an antibacterial spectrum similar to that of its parent compound although it is slightly more effective against sensitive bacteria on a weight basis. Absorption from the jejunum is rapid, and peak serum concentrations are obtained within 1 hour; these approximate 2 to 3 μg. per milliliter after the ingestion of 150 to 300 mg. Excretion is somewhat more rapid than for lincomycin, and serum levels are usually not measurable 8 hours after ingestion. Clinical trials with this drug are continuing, and it would appear that this drug is essentially equivalent to lincomycin. Some recent studies in vitro using clindamycin have indicated that it may be more active against anaerobic organisms than other antibiotics presently in use. Although several of these surveys have been carried out, there has not yet been sufficient clinical experience with this drug in anaerobic infections to recommend it unequivocally.

VANCOMYCIN

This is a bactericidal agent active only against gram-positive cocci. Its only clinical application at this time appears to be in the treatment of severe infections due to methicillin-resistant staphylococci and perhaps enterococci. Vancomycin is not absorbed from the alimentary tract and causes pain and necrosis when given intramuscularly. Administration is, therefore, always intravenous and over a five-minute period. One gram every 12 hours will give adequate blood levels against most staphylococci. It does not enter the cerebrospinal fluid or bile, and about 90% is excreted in the urine. Azotemia is a relative contraindication to its use, and vancomycin should not be employed in patients who have recently been exposed to other ototoxic or nephrotoxic agents.

A clinical use to which vancomycin is particularly well suited is the treatment of staphylococcal enterocolitis. Since the drug is not absorbed, 0.5 gm. in water or juice every 6 hours will give favorable results. Vancomycin is also finding increasing use in severe infections caused by methicillin-resistant staphylococci. It is, at this writing, the only effective bactericidal agent against the methicillin-resistant staphylococcus. Other work has shown that vancomycin may be an acceptable alternate to penicillin and streptomycin in the treatment of endocarditis caused by the enterococcus [15]. The number of patients treated thus far is small, however, and final judgment must be withheld until more experience has been accumulated. Synergism of vancomycin and streptomycin has been demonstrated in vivo [16], and this combination may ultimately be of value in persons unable to tolerate penicillin, although the toxicity will probably be high.

REFERENCES

1. Douthwaite, A. H., and Trafford, J. A. A new synthetic penicillin. *Brit. Med. J.* 2:687, 1960.
2. Steward, G. T., Harrison, P. M., and Holt, R. J. Microbiological studies on sodium 6-(2, 6-dimethoxylbenzamido) penicillanate monohydrate (BRL 1241) in vitro and in patients. *Brit. Med. J.* 2:694, 1960.
3. Douthwaite, A. H., Trafford, J. A. P., McGill, D. A. F., and Evans, I. E. Methicillin. *Brit. Med. J.* 2:6, 1961.
4. Hewitt, W. L. Penicillins: A review of strategy and tactics. *J.A.M.A.* 185:264, 1963.
5. McElfresh, A. E., and Huang, N. N. Bone-marrow depression resulting from the administration of methicillin. *New Eng. J. Med.* 266:246, 1962.
6. Klein, J. O., and Finland, M. The new penicillins. *New Eng. J. Med.* 269:1019, 1963.
7. Benner, E. J. The Cephalosporin Antibiotics. In B. M. Kagan (Ed.), *Antimicrobial Therapy.* Philadelphia: Saunders, 1970.
8. Perkins, R. L., Saslaw, S., and Hackett, J. Cephaloridine and cephalothin: Comparative *in vitro* evaluation. *Amer. J. Med. Sci.* 253:293, 1967.
9. Perkins, R. L., Carlisle, H. N., and Saslaw, S. Cephalexin: *In vitro* bacterial susceptibility, absorption in volunteers, and antibacterial activity of sera and urine. *Amer. J. Med. Sci.* 256:122, 1968.
10. Griffith, R. S. Comparison of bacteriostatic and bactericidal activity of penicillin, erythromycin, tetracycline, and chloramphenicol in human serum. *J. Lab. Clin. Med.* 56:820, 1960.

11. Kohlstaedt, K. G. Propionyl erythromycin ester lauryl sulfate and jaundice. *J.A.M.A.* 178:89, 1961.
12. Robinson, M. M. Antibiotics increase incidence of hepatitis. *J.A.M.A.* 178:89, 1961.
13. Rasch, J. R., and Mogabgab, W. J. *Mycoplasma pneumoniae* pneumonia: Efficacy of erythromycin, tetracycline, and demethylchlortetracycline in young adults. *Clin. Res.* 14:343, 1966.
14. Kaplan, K., Chew, W. H., and Weinstein, L. Microbiological, pharmacological, and clinical studies of lincomycin. *Amer. J. Med. Sci.* 250:137, 1965.
15. Friedberg, C. K., Rosen, K., and Bienstock, P. Vancomycin therapy for enterococcal and streptococcus viridans endocarditis. *Arch. Intern. Med.* 122:134, 1968.
16. Mandell, G. L., Lindsey, E., and Hook, E. W. Synergism of vancomycin and streptomycin for enterococci. *Amer. J. Med. Sci.* 259:346, 1970.

3 / MODIFICATION OF ANTIBIOTIC REGIMENS IN RENAL FAILURE

J. Joseph Marr

THE COMPLEXITY of antimicrobial therapy has increased as the number of new drugs and analogues of older agents has grown. The clinical practice of medicine has also been complicated by the necessity of using potentially toxic drugs in patients with diseases of the liver, kidney, or both. The current guidelines for drug administration to patients with these diseases are somewhat confusing, and there are many clinical studies, some of which are conflicting. The effect of dialysis, either peritoneal or hemodialysis, is only partly understood. Clinical guidelines also suffer from the lack of methods for accurate and rapid measurement of serum drug levels, and there is inadequate information regarding the activation of alternate pathways for drug metabolism when renal failure has supervened. Despite these flaws, it is possible to provide the clinician with approximate guidelines for adjustment of antibiotic dosage in uremia, recognizing that there will be a considerable variation among patients.

The absorption, distribution, and metabolism of a drug are reflected in the serum concentration of the agent in question. The absorption will vary in an unpredictable manner from individual to individual, and it is this variation that produces the wide range of dose-effect relationships among patients on a given therapeutic agent. For many drugs, the relation between the amount administered and the resulting concentration in the body is unpredictable. However, the intensity of the pharmacologic action generally correlates well with

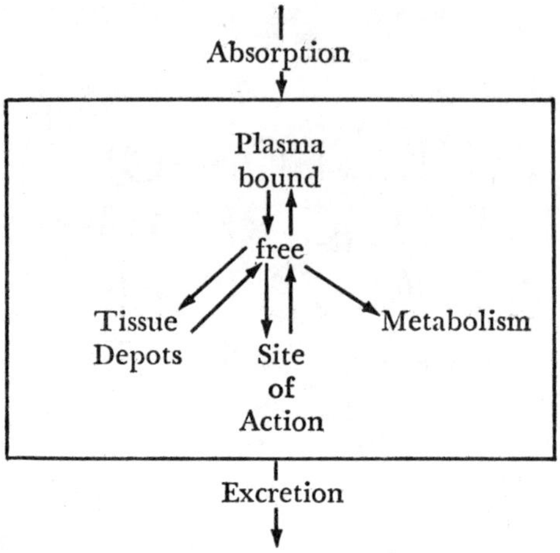

FIGURE 3-1 / Factors affecting the concentration of a drug in the serum.

the concentration of free drug finally obtained in the serum. As shown in Figure 3-1, the free concentration of the drug in the serum is dependent upon a multiplicity of factors. Redistribution of the agent to other tissues and accumulation in storage depots may be of some importance, particularly with the non-ionized or lipid-soluble drugs. Thus serum concentration, which is translated into pharmacologic effect, is in a dynamic steady-state equilibrium.

The length of time during which a drug exerts its effect is largely determined by its rate of inactivation and excretion. In conceptualizing the problems of drug administration to individuals with renal failure, one must assume a steady-state concentration of the agent in the plasma and define excretion of the drug as the rate-limiting step. Although this approach may lack the appeal of the controlled pharmacologic experiment, it nonetheless has direct clinical application and has been shown to be more than adequate under many and diverse circumstances. Since the major extrarenal site of drug excretion and inactivation is the liver, uremic patients with liver disease or jaundice will require markedly reduced dosages of all drugs and actual measurements of the concentrations in the serum may be necessary. An even greater reduction in dosage may be necessary in patients who are in shock or who are likely to have diminished renal and hepatic blood flow. This discussion assumes normal or nearly normal hepatic and circulatory functions.

The excretion of a drug may be measured as the decrease in serum concentration with time; this is usually a hyperbolic function, the slope of which at any particular time is a reflection of the serum concentration. Although the overall rate at which a drug is excreted

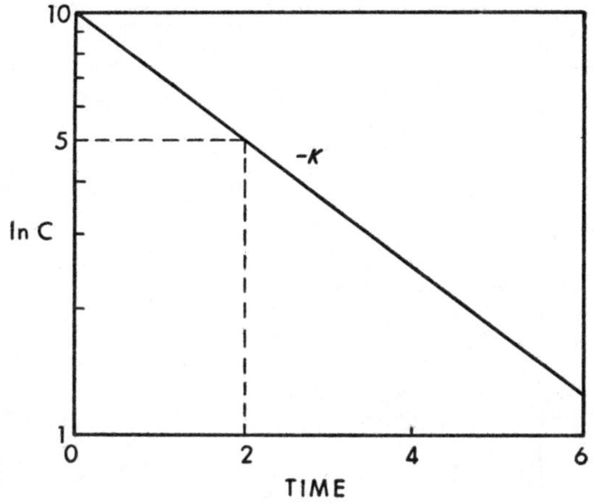

FIGURE 3-2 / Relationship of the logarithm of concentration to time.

depends upon its concentration, the fractional rate is not related to concentration, so that the logarithm of the serum concentration may be plotted as a linear function of time with a slope equal to K (Fig. 3-2). The value of this plot is evident, since the half-life of the drug may be easily calculated. The slope $(-K)$ is a constant and is determined by all of the conditions shown in Figure 3-1. A mere glance at this figure will be enough to convince one that this constant must be most inconstant. It is a reflection of the rate of excretion of a given agent from the plasma by the kidney and is dependent upon the status of the renal function at that time. Since the slope is a constant, at a given level of renal function the half-life $(T_{1/2})$ is *independent* of the concentration of the drug in the plasma. This is illustrated in Figure 3-3. As renal failure increases, the constant will increase proportionally and the serum concentration of the drug will decrease more slowly. This will be reflected in a longer half-life for the agent under consideration. This is illustrated in Figure 3-4. The corollary to this is that since the half-life is a constant at a given degree of renal function, one may either change the interval of administration of a drug or the amount of drug administered in that same interval to obtain a desired plasma concentration. Most experimental work, which has been done in patients with varying creatinine clearances (C_{CR}), has used normal doses of antibiotics to determine the half-lives of these agents. Thus it is easier clinically to employ normal doses and lengthen the intervals between these doses, although the reverse has been done with respect to dosage schedules for the cardiac glycosides.

In caring for a given patient with uremia, one must first esti-

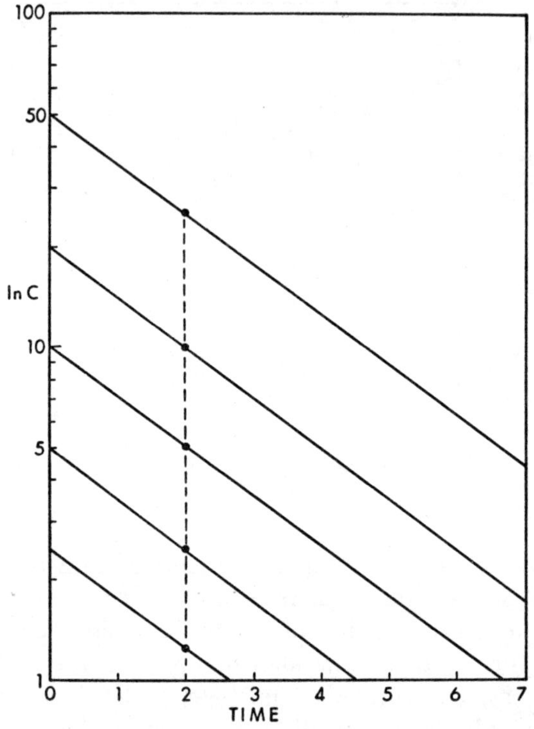

FIGURE 3-3 / Relationship of the logarithm of concentration to half-life.

mate the extent of renal failure in a manner which is reproducible from day to day. This would mean that a creatinine clearance should be done whenever possible and that a serum creatinine determination should be done at least. Blood urea nitrogen determinations, although they can be used, are less valid because they will vary with the state of hydration and the state of nutrition and may be somewhat less reproducible. Persons with a decreased creatinine clearance but a normal serum creatinine can usually receive normal antibiotic dosages. One also must determine the extent of concomitant liver disease. Although repeated creatinine clearances are the preferred method for monitoring alterations in glomerular filtration rate, it is possible to measure the serum creatinine initially at the time of the clearance study and to compare subsequent determinations with it in order to ascertain changes in the glomerular filtration rate. For example, if the creatinine clearance is 50% of normal when the individual's creatinine is 2 mg. per 100 ml., a subsequent serum creatinine of 4 mg. per 100 ml. would mean that the creatinine clearance had fallen to 25% of normal or

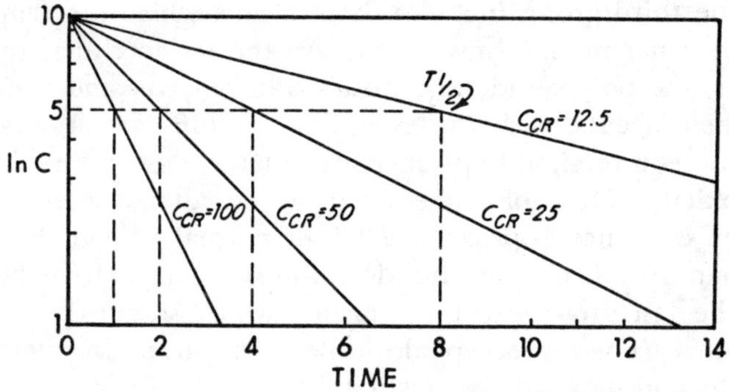

FIGURE 3-1 / Relationship of creatinine clearance to half-life. *In C* = natural logarithm of concentration; C_{CR} = creatinine clearance.

had decreased by half. Since most drugs excreted by the kidney are excreted in a roughly linear relation to the creatinine clearance, the dose interval may be determined from either the creatinine clearance or the serum creatinine, since the latter bears a linear relationship to the former. Drugs are usually given as a loading dose and then as normal maintenance doses with lengthening dose intervals as the creatinine clearance declines.

GENERAL GUIDELINES

The chemotherapeutic agents may be divided into four groups on the basis of their usefulness in patients with renal insufficiency. This separation implies nothing regarding mode of action or chemical similarity, but serves only as a guide to potential toxicity when used in the presence of uremia.

The first group of agents contains those drugs which are excreted primarily by nonrenal mechanisms. These include chlortetracycline, erythromycin, chloramphenicol, chloroquine, amphotericin B, and isoniazid. They can generally be used in uremia with no modification in dosage. Inactive metabolites may accumulate but are nontoxic and can generally be disregarded. The next group of agents includes those antibiotics which are cleared by both renal and extrarenal mechanisms. These include the penicillins, the cephalosporins, and lincomycin. These require only slight modification in dose interval, even when the creatinine clearance falls below 10 ml. per minute. A notable exception is cephaloridine, which is excreted primarily through renal mechanisms and in the presence of uremia is very nephrotoxic. It should not be used in renal failure.

The third group includes those agents which are removed primarily by renal mechanisms. These are the tetracyclines, the aminoglycosides, the polypeptide antibiotics, vancomycin, and sulfisoxazole. All of these agents, with the exception of sulfisoxazole, are nephrotoxic and require significant increases in the dose interval to avoid nephrotoxicity. Most of these need to be altered even when the creatinine clearance approaches 50% of normal. When the clearance is less than 10 ml. per minute, dose intervals are extremely long.

The last group are those agents which should be avoided in renal failure. These are cephaloridine, nitrofurantoin, methenamine mandelate, and para-aminosalicylic acid.

Agents Excreted by Both Renal and Nonrenal Mechanisms

These are generally of low toxicity and can be used with relative impunity in azotemic patients. Dose-interval modification for uremia is shown in Table 3-1.

Penicillins. Under normal conditions penicillin G and the semisynthetic penicillins are excreted primarily via the kidney. Approximately 10% of penicillin G is eliminated by glomerular filtration and 90% by tubular excretion. Renal clearance therefore approximates the total renal plasma flow. Although the semisynthetic penicillins are excreted in the same manner, they are also excreted to a moderate extent in the bile. This is particularly true of ampicillin, although it is subject to enterohepatic recirculation and its ultimate excretion is via the kidney. Carbenicillin is excreted in the same manner as penicillin G. It should be remembered that 10 gm. of carbenicillin contain 45 mEq. of sodium; this may be important in treating persons with renal impairment.

Cephalosporins. These are all derivatives of 7-aminocephalosporanic acid and as such are comparable to the extended-spectrum penicillins. Cephalothin exhibits a larger relative volume distribution and longer plasma half-life than do the phenoxyalkyl penicillins. About 70 to 80% is excreted unchanged in the urine via tubular secretion. Part of the agent is transformed into the O-desacetyl metabolite which is biologically inactive and is excreted in the urine together with the active compound. Cephaloridine is nephrotoxic and should be avoided in the presence of renal failure.

Cephalexin is one of the newer members of the cephalosporin group, and it has the advantage that oral administration achieves excellent absorption and appreciable serum and urine concentrations. It is useful as an agent for treating infections in ambulatory patients and as a continuing medication after initial therapy with a parenteral cephalosporin. Its absorption is independent of renal function, and no

TABLE 3-1 / Dose-Interval Modifications for Agents of Low Toxicity

Drug	Maintenance Dose Interval (hr.) Based on Creatinine Clearance (ml./min.)				Modification for Dialysis	
	100	80–50	50–10	< 10	Hemodialysis	Peritoneal
Penicillins						
Penicillin G	q8h	8	8	12	None	None
Oxacillin[a]	q6h	8	8	10–12	None	None
Methicillin	q4h	8	8	8–12	None	None
Ampicillin	q6h	8	8	12		Add 50 mg./L. dialysis fluid
Carbenicillin[b]	q4h	4	6–12	12	Add 2 gm. after dialysis	Add to dialysis fluid at desired serum concentration
Cephalosporins						
Cephalothin	q6h	6	6	8–12	One dose before and q4h during hemodialysis	Add to fluid at desired serum levels
Cephalexin	q4–6h	4–6	8–10	36–64	Give 500 mg. before and after dialysis	Add to fluid at desired serum levels

[a] Applies to other isoxazolyl penicillins; biliary excretion increases during renal failure.
[b] Assumes that infection is extraurinary, and 4 to 5 gm. doses are required.
Modified from Washington University Department of Medicine *Manual of Medical Therapeutics,* 20th ed., M. G. Rosenfeld (Ed.), Boston: Little, Brown, 1971, based on W. M. Bennett et al. [1], P. A. Greenberg and J. P. Sanford [2], C. M. Kunin [3].

modification of dose is necessary at creatinine clearances greater than 30 ml. per minute. In patients who are undergoing hemodialysis, cephalexin is absorbed more rapidly. This may be due to changes in percentage of blood flow to the gastrointestinal tract, although the specific reason is not clear.

The persistance of cephalexin in the serum of patients with severe renal failure and the exponential decay rates suggest that cephalexin in vivo is handled differently from cephalothin. The relation between the half-life and renal function and the behavior of cephalexin and of cephaloridine in dialysis suggests an in vivo similarity in handling of these two cephalosporins.

Erythromycin and Lincomycin. About 2 to 5% of orally administered erythromycin is excreted in the urine; about 15% is detectable after intravenous infusion. Erythromycin is concentrated in the liver and excreted in an active form in the bile. Lincomycin is pharmacologically and therapeutically similar to erythromycin; its mode of excretion and toxicity are likewise comparable. The recently introduced drug clindamycin (7-chlorolincomycin) is essentially the same as lincomycin. Both of these drugs may be used in the presence of renal failure and usually do not require a reduction in dosage. They are not dialyzed significantly by either route.

Chloramphenicol. This agent is inactivated primarily in the liver, and the nontoxic glucuronide is rapidly excreted in the urine. Over a 24-hour period about 90% of an orally administered dose is excreted in the urine. About 10% is in the biologically active form, and the remainder is a hydrolysis product and the glucuronic acid conjugate. The unaltered antibiotic is eliminated by glomerular filtration and the inactive degradation products primarily by tubular secretion. In the presence of renal insufficiency, the plasma half-life of the biologically active drug is not significantly prolonged but that of the conjugated inactive form is markedly extended. Because of this fact, the regimen for persons with kidney disease is the same as that for normal subjects. Although the rate at which chloramphenicol is conjugated with glucuronic acid may be reduced in individuals with hepatic failure, the overall metabolism is essentially normal. Nevertheless, the administration of chloramphenicol in the presence of liver disease frequently results in depression of erythropoiesis. Chloramphenicol is not removed significantly by either method of dialysis.

Agents Excreted Primarily by Renal Mechanisms

Most of these chemotherapeutic agents are toxic when they are allowed to accumulate in the blood. Consequently, their use should be avoided in patients with renal failure unless the clinical situation

TABLE 3-2 / Dose-Interval Modifications for Agents with Significant Toxicity

	Maintenance Dose Interval (hr.) Based on Creatinine Clearance (ml./min.)				Modification for Dialysis	
Drug	100	80–50	50–10	< 10	Hemodialysis	Peritoneal
Streptomycin	q12h	24	24–72	72–96	Add 250 mg. at end of each dialysis	
Kanamycin	q8h	24	24–72	72–96	Give 7 mg./kg. after every other dialysis	Add to fluid at desired serum levels
Gentamicin[a]	q8h	8–12	12–24	48	Give 80 mg. after each dialysis	
Vancomycin	q12h	24–72	72–240	240	None	
Tetracycline	q6h	12	48	72–96	None	
Colistimethate	q12h	24	36–60	60–92	None	2 mg./kg./day during dialysis

[a] Based on a dosage schedule 1 mg. per kilogram of body weight.

Modified from Washington University Department of Medicine *Manual of Medical Therapeutics,* 20th ed., M. G. Rosenfeld (Ed.), Boston: Little, Brown, 1971, based on W. M. Bennett et al. [1], P. A. Greenberg and J. P. Sanford [2], C. M. Kunin [3].

and microbial sensitivity patterns dictate otherwise. The dose-interval modifications for these drugs are given in Table 3-2.

Tetracyclines. The tetracyclines must be administered with caution in individuals with renal impairment, although there are differences among these antibiotics with respect to their persistence in the blood and in the amounts recovered in the urine in persons with renal insufficiency. For example, in azotemia tetracycline persists in the blood for an extended period of time while chlortetracycline is excreted almost as it is in normal individuals. The extent to which the tetracyclines are excreted in the urine in the presence of renal insufficiency is in the following order of decreasing amount: oxytetracycline, tetracycline, demethylchlortetracycline, chlortetracycline. Table 3-2 gives the dosage modification for generic tetracycline in persons with renal insufficiency. This drug is the best studied of all of the tetracyclines and is therefore preferred for use in persons with renal failure. There is little information regarding the metabolism of the other tetracyclines in renal insufficiency, and their use is best avoided.

A recently introduced tetracycline, doxycycline, is a semisynthetic tetracycline analogue. It differs somewhat from other tetracyclines by its nearly complete absorption after oral administration, and it may be given with either food or milk. It has prolonged in vivo antibacterial activity which persists for about 24 hours; thus it may be given once a day or only twice a day at most. Clinical studies have indicated that it differs from other tetracyclines by its relatively low renal clearance, and excessive serum accumulation does not occur in persons with impaired renal function. This would imply that metabolic pathways not normally utilized for this drug are activated in the presence of renal failure so that the serum concentration remains unchanged. The urinary excretion of doxycycline falls proportionately with the creatinine clearance and becomes negligible in severe renal insufficiency. Fecal excretion of this drug in uremic patients is found to be at or below normal levels. Other studies of anuric patients have indicated that there is no appreciable change in the half-life of this drug with hemodialysis. Although the initial clinical experience with this drug is most encouraging, judgment regarding its use in patients with renal impairment should be held in abeyance until more experience has been accumulated.

Aminoglycosides. One must be extremely circumspect in administering these agents to an individual with renal insufficiency. In patients with anuria, blood levels may remain high for many days and permanent ototoxicity is very common. About 50 to 60% of a parenterally administered dose of streptomycin appears in the urine in the first 24 hours. The rate of renal clearance of streptomycin in man is about 30% lower than the glomerular filtration rate. Kanamycin is primarily filtered by the glomeruli, and about 50 to 80% is recoverable in the urine in a 24-hour period following injection. Gentamicin is cleared most rapidly—in about 6 to 8 hours.

Of the aminoglycosides, neomycin is perhaps the most toxic, producing tubular damage at doses only two to three times the therapeutic dose; it will not be discussed further. Kanamycin is intermediate in toxicity, producing damage at three to ten times the therapeutic dose; streptomycin has only mild renal toxicity, requiring about twenty times the therapeutic dose. Gentamicin appears to have very little nephrotoxicity, although experimental work indicates that it probably is of the order of streptomycin. Nevertheless, because of their propensity to cause renal tubular damage, these drugs are not given in combination, even in the presence of normal renal function. Vancomycin achieves much higher concentrations in the blood of persons with renal insufficiency, since about 80% of an injected dose is excreted by the kidneys under normal conditions. This drug should, therefore, be avoided in persons with renal insufficiency.

The aminoglycosides have been among the best studied chemotherapeutic agents in persons with renal insufficiency. The recommendations given in Table 3-2 represent a synthesis of much of this work. However, there are additional papers which may be consulted which enable one to base the dose on the serum creatinine and to calculate the half-life therefrom. The studies by Cutler and coworkers [4, 5] using kanamycin and gentamicin are recommended.

Polymyxins. These are excreted by the kidneys and possess a significant nephrotoxicity. Polymyxin B appears to be somewhat more toxic than polymyxin E (colistin). For this reason, only the latter will be described. The methane sulfonate salt (colistimethate) is hydrolyzed to yield colistin in the tissues. The salt releases the antibiotic slowly from injection sites, thereby damping fluctuations in serum concentration. The height and duration of plasma concentration are related to the degree of renal insufficiency, and hemodialysis does not reduce the quantity of this drug in the circulation of uremic patients.

Agents Avoided in Renal Insufficiency

Nitrofurantoin, methenamine mandelate (Mandelamine), and paraaminosalicylic acid should be avoided in persons with renal failure. Unlike the other cephalosporins, cephaloridine should not be used in persons with renal insufficiency since it is excreted primarily by tubular secretory mechanisms which are apparently not used for cephalothin and cephalexin. As mentioned above, vancomycin should be avoided in persons with renal insufficiency; however, due to the fact that it is occasionally required for treatment of penicillin-resistant staphylococci or perhaps the enterococci, it has been included in Table 3-2.

TREATMENT OF URINARY TRACT INFECTIONS IN PATIENTS WITH UREMIA

The treatment of urinary tract infections in persons with uremia is a particularly difficult problem, since the problem of toxicity due to increased serum levels of antibiotics is then compounded by the additional problem of ineffective levels of antibiotics in the urine. An antibiotic for the treatment of patients with urinary tract infections and uremia should be one that is rapidly excreted into the urine, slowly metabolized, nontoxic in high concentrations in the blood, and that has a rather broad spectrum of activity. At this time the best agents are probably ampicillin and cephalexin. Both of these may be administered orally, both appear in the urine in high concentrations, even with a creatinine clearance of less than 10 ml. per minute, and there is no evidence of further renal toxicity as the drug is given.

Although nitrofurantoin has a rapid clearance, it is even more rapidly inactivated by other mechanisms in renal failure and does not appear in the urine. Moreover, even the small quantities of this drug which appear in the serum are highly toxic. The sulfonamides, although excreted primarily through renal mechanisms, usually will not give an adequate effect because sulfonamide-resistant organisms are common in patients with recurrent urinary tract infections. Sulphadimidine is a drug which has been reported to be cleared as rapidly by severely uremic patients as normal subjects and to give equally high concentrations in the urine, although more recent data would indicate that the drug does accumulate in uremic patients. Ultimately this may prove useful in treating sulfonamide-sensitive organisms in uremic patients. At this time the drugs most likely to be of value in this clinical situation are ampicillin and cephalexin.

REFERENCES

1. Bennett, W. M., Singer, I., and Coggins, C. H. A practical guide to drug usage in adult patients with impaired renal function. *J.A.M.A.* 214:1468, 1970.
2. Greenberg, P. A., and Sanford, J. P. Removal and absorption of antibiotics in patients with renal failure undergoing peritoneal dialysis. *Ann. Intern. Med.* 66:465, 1967.

3. Kunin, C. M. A guide to use of antibiotics in patients with renal disease. *Ann. Intern. Med.* 67:151, 1967.
4. Cutler, R. E., Gyselynck, A. M., Fleet, W. P., and Forrey, A. W. Correlation of serum creatinine concentration and gentamicin half-life. *J.A.M.A.* 219:1037, 1972.
5. Cutler, R. E., and Orme, B. M. Correlation of serum creatinine concentration and kanamycin half-life. *J.A.M.A.* 209:539, 1969.
6. Fischer, E. Renal excretion of sulphadimidine in normal and uremic subjects. *Lancet* 2:210, 1972.

4 / PULMONARY INFECTIONS

Paul M. Southern, Jr.

THIS CHAPTER will review some of the major features of acute and subacute infectious disorders of the bronchopulmonary system, including acute infectious bronchitis, bronchopneumonia, lobar pneumonia, putrid lung abscess, and certain other related clinical syndromes. It will not include a discussion of chronic bronchitis or of the chronic granulomatous infections of the lung, such as pulmonary tuberculosis and infections by atypical mycobacteria. Emphasis will be placed on diagnostic procedures, microbiologic etiologies, and antimicrobial chemotherapy.

GENERAL DIAGNOSTIC PROCEDURES

Of all the specimens routinely handled in a clinical microbiology laboratory, none is so often misused as the sputum specimen. It is well known that the mouth and pharynx are the site of colonization by a myriad of microorganisms. Some of these, such as the pneumococcus, the meningococcus, and various gram-negative bacilli, are potentially pathogenic organisms but may be present in the throat of normal individuals who are permanent or transient carriers of the organisms. Sputum which is expectorated through this contaminated site would be expected to reflect on culture the organisms which reside in the mouth and pharynx. On the other hand, because of overgrowth of a culture by normal upper airway flora, more fastidious organisms, which may be responsible for an infection in the lung, may fail to grow or be recognized on culture. With these factors in mind, the following diagnostic procedures are recommended in evaluating individuals suspected of having pulmonary infections.

Sputum Smear. Frequently more valuable information is derived by careful microscopical examination of a sputum smear than by culture of the same specimen. In most instances, gram and methylene blue stains of sputum should be done; depending upon the type of organism suspected, other more specialized stains may be indicated. The smear should be evaluated for the presence of epithelial squames, which is an indication the specimen is saliva rather than sputum. Specimens containing large numbers of squamous epithelial cells should not be cultured. The presence of mucoid material and polymorphonuclear leukocytes is helpful in establishing whether an infectious process is likely. Furthermore, the smear should be examined for the presence of bacteria, their morphology, and their site (extracellular, intracellular, or both). Useful clues to the etiology of an infectious process may be derived from the morphology of organisms seen.

Sputum Culture. As indicated, routine culture of sputum is fraught with many difficulties. Because of this, certain variations and modifications of the usual techniques are indicated. Sputum washing techniques may be valuable in excluding surface contamination of a specimen by oropharyngeal organisms. A variety of methods can be used. For example, place a large portion of a purulent specimen on sterile surgical gauze in the bottom of a wire tea strainer. Place a second layer of sterile surgical gauze over the top of the specimen and expose this to a jet of cold tap water for ten seconds. The material remaining is then cultured either quantitatively or semiquantitatively with a calibrated loop. Other measures which may be of value include accurate quantitative sputum cultures and sputum homogenization. The latter may be performed with sputum and saline or with sputum and acetylcysteine in conjunction with quantitative culture technique. Detailed descriptions of these procedures are available in the literature.

Transtracheal Aspiration. This method of obtaining sputum for culture avoids the contamination of the upper airway and provides an accurate assessment of the flora present in the lung. In addition, one may culture a specimen obtained transtracheally for anaerobic organisms, which cannot be done with expectorated sputum because of the large numbers of anaerobes which reside normally in the mouth and pharynx.

A few precautions must be taken in performing transtracheal aspiration, and a certain modicum of skill is necessary to master the technique. Transtracheal aspiration is carried out by hyperextending the patient's neck over a pillow so that the first three or four tracheal rings are easily felt. The entire procedure should be done in an aseptic manner with the anterior portion of the neck cleansed with surgical soap and an iodine solution. The trachea may be entered through the cricothyroid membrane or at a site between the first few rings below the thyroid cartilage. If the latter is chosen as the point of entry, one should go to the left side of the midline since about 10% of persons have a thyroidea ima artery. After instillation of lidocaine into the area, an 8-inch medium polyethylene catheter is passed into the trachea and then directed into the appropriate main-stem bronchus. The needle is removed from the neck, and the catheter is left in place. Two or 3 ml. of sterile saline is then instilled into the bronchus and aspirated. The catheter is removed, and a bandage may be placed over the puncture site. When the neck is returned to the normal position, the needle track will be obliterated.

Reported complications of transtracheal aspiration include hemoptysis, localized subcutaneous emphysema, mediastinal emphysema, subcutaneous abscess, cardiac arrhythmias, and hypoxia. With careful attention to technique, patient selection, and monitoring, these can be avoided in most instances. Serious complications are very infrequent.

Bronchoscopy. While bronchoscopy is frequently useful in establishing effective drainage and in visually identifying various lesions, culture of material obtained at bronchoscopy is also to some extent subject to contamination by oropharyngeal organisms. For this reason it is less useful as a source of culture material than is transtracheal aspiration.

Bronchial Brush Biopsy. This procedure, usually done via a transtracheal approach, is quite helpful in obtaining material for cytologic and microbiologic evaluation. It is ordinarily done under fluoroscopic control, enabling accurate placement of the catheter tip in close proximity to the lesion in question, and one may often penetrate cavitary lesions by this method. Secretions obtained by this means can be treated in the same fashion as those obtained by direct transtracheal aspiration.

Percutaneous Transthoracic Aspiration. Material can be obtained for smear, culture, and cytologic examination via direct aspiration from lung parenchyma. This method is applicable to patients with peripherally placed pulmonary lesions and in those with pleural adhesions or pleural effusions or both. It is helpful in the latter circumstance to combine the procedure with study of pleural fluid and with pleural biopsy. Materials obtained by this method are quite satisfactory for microbiologic examination. Complications include hemorrhage, pneumothorax, and occasional cardiac arrhythmias. The procedure is contraindicated in the presence of pulmonary hypertension, bullous pulmonary lesions, and hemorrhagic diathesis.

Surgical and Postmortem Lung Cultures. Materials carefully obtained by sterile technique at surgery or postmortem examination are quite helpful in determining the microbial etiology of pulmonary infectious processes. Lung biopsy is frequently the only successful method of making a correct diagnosis in many infections, particularly in the case of *Pneumocystis carinii.*

SPECIFIC ETIOLOGIC CATEGORIES

Gram-Positive Bacteria

Diplococcus pneumoniae. The pneumococcus, a lancet-shaped, gram-positive coccus usually occurring in pairs or short chains, is responsible for a large percentage of all primary bacterial pneumonias. Most disease-causing pneumococci belong to the lower numbered capsular types, with eleven types accounting for 75 to 85% of all pneumococcal pulmonary disease (I–V, VII, VIII, XII, XIV, XIX, and XXIII). Although pneumococci may be normal inhabitants of the nose or throat, they may be responsible for numerous infections, including pneumonia, meningitis, otitis media, arthritis, pericarditis, peritonitis, and other localized infections. Pneumonia is the most prevalent of these infections. It is debatable whether pneumococci ever cause primary bronchopneumonia; however, other types of inflammatory lesions, such as interstitial pneumonia, may become secondarily infected with pneumococci and expressed in the form of bronchopneumonia.

Classic pneumococcal lobar pneumonia, although more prominent in males and at the extremes of age, occurs in all races, both sexes, and all ages. Association with a nonspecific or viral upper respiratory infection is not unusual. Although the exact pathogenesis is not clear, it is likely related to aspiration of a small-particle aerosol, either from an endogenous source or airborne.

The illness itself is usually heralded by the appearance of one or more of the major triad of symptoms: chills, hemoptysis, and pleurisy. If none of these symptoms is present, a bacterial etiology is indicated by a sudden worsening during the course of an upper respiratory infection, with dyspnea or heightened cough. The inflammatory reaction is generally acute, with alveolar exudation in a segmental or lobar distribution. Spread through contiguous segments and lobes is not uncommon. Bloodstream invasion also occurs, indicating a need for blood cultures in all individuals with acute pneumonia. A typical individual with pneumococcal pneumonia has one to three chills and pleuritic pain of the conventional variety. At times the pain may be referred to other areas, such as the neck, shoulders, or abdomen. The latter presentation is responsible for a significant number of individuals with pneumococcal lobar pneumonia being diagnosed as having an acute surgical abdomen and mistakenly being subjected to laparotomy.

Sputum is usually pink, but varying degrees of blood-streaked or grossly bloody sputum are not uncommon. Temperature usually rises abruptly to 102° to 105°F., and fever is generally present throughout the early course of the disease, ordinarily ending abruptly with a crisis or by rapid lysis. In the absence of multilobar consolidation, dyspnea is usually the result of pleuritic pain. Obstructive dyspnea is uncommon except in small infants and children.

The occurrence of physical findings suggestive of pleural effusion is uncommon early in the disease. However, a syndrome of pleural effusion at seven to ten days into the course of the illness, even in the face of appropriate antibiotic therapy, is not unusual. This may be associated with abrupt reappearance of pleuritic pain, fever, and leukocytosis. The pleural fluid is sterile, and the syndrome is not to be confused with empyema, which may occur in untreated individuals, in persons with inadequate therapy, or in whom normal host defense mechanisms may be impaired.

Chest films usually demonstrate segmental or lobar consolidation. Cavitation is unusual. Progression of roentgenographic abnormalities in the face of appropriate therapy is not unusual, and roentgenographic improvement may lag many days behind apparent clinical improvement. On the other hand, if films are taken during the first few hours to one day after the onset of clinical illness, no abnormality may be apparent. In a typical case of pneumococcal pneumonia the roentgenographic appearance is a useful confirmatory procedure, although similar syndromes may be caused by other bacterial and nonbacterial diseases.

Diagnostic studies indicated in suspected pneumococcal pneumonia include culture of respiratory secretions, blood cultures, sputum smears, and leukocyte counts. Occasionally leukemoid responses are seen. Leukopenia, when present, is a poor prognostic sign.

The antibacterial therapy of choice in uncomplicated pneumococcal lobar pneumonia is penicillin G in low doses (1.2 to 2.4

million units per day). In the individual with a history of penicillin sensitivity, erythromycin is the alternative agent of choice. Because of an incidence of tetracycline resistance in 4 to 5% of pneumococci, this agent should not be used in primary therapy of pneumonia. Individuals with underlying emphysema, pulmonary fibrosis, diabetes mellitus, alcoholism, or other derangements of host defense mechanisms should probably be treated initially with agents effective against pneumococci, group A streptococci, *Klebsiella pneumoniae, Haemophilus influenzae,* and *Staphylococcus aureus* until it is clearly established that the etiology of the infection is pneumococcal. Five to seven days of therapy is usually adequate for uncomplicated pneumococcal lobar pneumonia.

Streptococcus pyogenes. Streptococcus pyogenes is a gram-positive coccus that characteristically grows in chains, particularly in liquid media. On blood agar, it produces zones of complete (clear, β) hemolysis. By serologic methods, groups A through N may be distinguished. Most human disease is related to group A, which can be further subdivided into many M types. Less commonly, groups B, C, D, E, F, and G may cause disease in human beings.

Streptococcal disease usually occurs as tonsillitis or pharyngitis or as cutaneous disease such as impetigo, erysipelas, or scarlet fever. Pneumonia is a relatively uncommon manifestation. However, in children, especially following respiratory diseases such as pertussis, measles, and other viral respiratory illnesses, streptococcal pneumonia is a relatively common complication. In adults, secondary streptococcal pneumonia may be seen as a complication of influenza, and it has been described in epidemics in military recruit populations. The occurrence of pharyngitis, cervical adenitis, mastoiditis, or cutaneous manifestations might indicate infection due to group A streptococci. The early process is usually bronchopneumonic but may progress to lobar consolidation. Early development of a pleural effusion or empyema is characteristic.

Streptococcal infections, including pneumonia, may be complicated by the development of certain nonsuppurative pulmonary conditions. These include rheumatic pneumonia, glomerulonephritis with pulmonary edema (which may be mistaken for bronchopneumonia), and poststreptococcal erythema multiforme with hilar lymph node involvement.

Therapy of streptococcal pneumonia is similar to that described for pneumococcal pneumonia, except that its duration should be extended to ten days in order to prevent late nonsuppurative complications.

Staphylococcus aureus. Most pathogenic staphylococci are

classified as *S. aureus.* These are large, gram-positive cocci, usually occurring in clusters and less frequently as individual organisms, pairs, or short chains. They may be further characterized by coagulase, deoxyribonuclease, and anaerobic mannitol fermentation. For epidemiologic purposes, strains are usually characterized by bacteriophage typing. *Staphylococcus epidermidis,* which is usually a skin commensal, is, under certain circumstances, capable of being a human pathogen.

Staphylococci may be transmitted via airborne dust and dry particles as well as by person-to-person or person-to-fomite routes. Many individuals (from 20 to 50% at different times) are carriers of staphylococci in their anterior nares, and many chronic carriers have periodic skin infections. Occasional individuals are perineal carriers of staphylococci.

Although the majority of staphylococcal disease is cutaneous, it may spread to become systemic from that site or it may involve the respiratory tract initially. In infants and children, tracheitis, bronchitis, and pneumonia occur particularly after viral respiratory illnesses and other virus diseases such as measles. On the other hand, adult staphylococcal pneumonia occurs largely following influenza or as a consequence of bacteremia. In the latter case, the pulmonary disease is characteristically an embolic process, with scattered abscesses appearing in the pulmonary parenchyma. This kind of pneumonic involvement may occur as a consequence of right-sided endocarditis, especially in drug addicts, in which case it may be due either to *S. aureus* or *epidermidis.* Staphylococci are characteristically histotoxic, and abscess formation and subsequent cavitation are common in staphylococcal pulmonary infections. Empyema is a frequent accompaniment of staphylococcal pulmonary disease. In children, the appearance of pneumatoceles is relatively common.

The radiographic appearance of staphylococcal pneumonia may be somewhat pleomorphic. Following other respiratory infections such as influenza, it may be widespread and bronchopneumonic in nature, but generally it is characterized by abscess formation and empyema.

Antimicrobial therapy of staphylococcal pneumonia is best accomplished with a penicillinase-resistant synthetic penicillin in high doses (8 to 12 gm. per day). In the event of penicillin sensitivity, alternative agents include vancomycin or possibly gentamicin or kanamycin (the last two agents should not be used unless the organism involved has been demonstrated to be sensitive to the drugs in vitro). Bacteriostatic agents such as lincomycin, erythromycin, or chloramphenicol should not be used as initial therapy for staphylococcal pneumonia. Adjunctive diagnostic and therapeutic measures may at times include bronchoscopy and drainage of abscesses or empyema. Antimicrobial therapy is usually required for a period of three to six weeks, depending upon the response and whether endocarditis is present.

Enterococcus. Occasionally enterococci (usually group D streptococci) are associated with pulmonary infections, usually as a consequence of septic embolization either from bacterial endocarditis or from an infected focus within the abdomen or pelvis. This type of pulmonary infection is usually manifested by pulmonary infarcts and subsequent abscess formation.

Gram-Negative Bacteria

Enterobacteriaceae. The family Enterobacteriaceae is composed of many genera, the most important of which are *Shigella, Salmonella, Klebsiella, Enterobacter, Serratia,* and *Proteus.* Probably all the enterobacteriaceae are capable of producing pulmonary infections under appropriate circumstances. The most frequent causes of primary pulmonary infection among these organisms are the klebsiellae. The most common pulmonary pathogen in this genus is *K. pneumoniae,* Friedländer's bacillus, which has a characteristic thick capsule.

Klebsiellae. These occur in normal persons, but the prevalence is low (1 to 4%). In hospitalized and ill patients this prevalence in pharyngeal cultures may increase to as high as 25%. It is likely that pulmonary infections arise from inhalation or aspiration of organisms residing in the oropharynx, particularly if the usual pulmonary microbial defense mechanisms (i.e., alveolar macrophages and mucociliary activity) are compromised. For this reason, *Klebsiella* pulmonary infections are frequently seen in certain types of patients, such as alcoholics, individuals with chronic obstructive pulmonary disease, and diabetics. Patients with primary *Klebsiella* pneumonia are predominantly males (80 to 90%), are middle-aged or older, and in many instances from predominantly black populations.

The pneumonia is similar in onset to pneumococcal pneumonia, with abrupt appearance of cough, sputum production, pleuritic chest pain, and chills. The onset may be preceded by an undifferentiated upper respiratory infection. The classic description of sputum in *Klebsiella* pneumonia is that of currant jelly, often a bright or brick red color. Patients are characteristically acutely ill, febrile, dyspneic, and cyanotic, and examination of the chest usually reveals signs of consolidation. Involvement of multiple lobes is not uncommon, with a predilection for upper lobes.

The chest roentgenogram is variable and may include massive lobar consolidation, multilobar involvement, abscess formation with large cavities, or multiple, small, thin-walled cavities, and bulging fissures. During resolution, residual parenchymal fibrosis is not uncommon. Laboratory features include leukocyte counts ranging from marked leukocytosis to marked leukopenia, the latter being a poor prognostic sign. Blood cultures are positive in a small percentage of patients. Complications include rapid destruction of pulmonary parenchyma with large cavity formation and residual fibrosis. Pneumothorax and pleural effusions are less common.

On the basis of in vitro susceptibility studies, klebsiellae are found to be susceptible in most cases to chloramphenicol, gentamicin, kanamycin, colistimethate, polymyxin B, and, to a lesser extent, cephalothin. In patients who are not seriously ill, gentamicin, kanamycin, or cephalothin may be used alone. However, in seriously ill patients, a combination of cephalothin and either kanamycin or gentamicin may be indicated. It is mandatory that measures be directed at maintenance of clear airways and adequate drainage of abscess cavities.

Virtually any of the enterobacteriaceae are capable of causing secondary pulmonary infections. These are frequently nosocomial infections and occur in patients with underlying conditions such as bronchial obstruction, chronic bronchitis, or emphysema, or after prolonged antibacterial therapy against gram-positive bacteria. Patients receiving steroids or other immunosuppressive agents and patients receiving frequent or continuous nebulization therapy with contaminated equipment or solutions are also at risk. Although organisms of this category usually do not produce primary pulmonary infections, the reports of Tillotson and Lerner point to such a possibility. Ordinarily the clinical setting is not sufficiently characteristic to allow an etiologic classification without microbiologic confirmation. The disease in the lung may be lobar or bronchopneumonic. Progression to abscess formation is not uncommon. All of these organisms have the capacity to produce necrotizing pulmonary lesions; the major problem in this regard is establishing the correct bacteriologic diagnosis.

Opportunistic Gram-Negative Bacilli. Organisms in this group include the genera *Achromobacter, Alcaligenes, Herellea, Mima,* and *Pseudomonas* among others. With certain exceptions, to be described below, pulmonary infections produced by these organisms are usually of the secondary or nosocomial variety. In recent years the prevalence of isolation of these organisms from pulmonary secretions has increased dramatically. This is in large part due to increased use of inhalation therapy incorporating reservoir nebulization, antimicrobial drugs in large quantities, corticosteroids, and immunosuppressive agents. In addition, diagnostic laboratories have improved in their abilities to identify these organisms. Because they are ubiquitous (especially in areas of high humidity and moisture content), they are quite common in many types of hospital environments. For this reason, isolation of the organism from sputum does not necessarily mean the patient is infected. This is an even greater problem in a patient with a tracheostomy, wherein multiple potential sources for contamination and colonization exist. For these reasons it is often difficult to assign an etiologic role to one of these organisms in a pulmonary infection in an individual patient.

These organisms are infrequently responsible for primary pulmonary infection, although occasional cases have been described, particularly in the instance of *P. aeruginosa*. Infections due to this organism may be either bacteremic or airborne in origin. In the former, necrotizing vascular involvement is common, but such involvement is less common in the airborne variety. In either case, a necrotizing pneumonia is not unusual. With all of these organisms, the clinical features are similar to those described above under Enterobacteriaceae. Empyema, bronchopleural fistula, and abscess formation are not uncommon. Clinical findings, such as physical examination, leukocyte counts, and chest radiographs, are not of great discriminatory assistance. Sputum cultures must be interpreted with caution, and the diagnosis frequently rests on sputum smear and a high index of clinical suspicion. Diagnosis by culture of empyema or pleural fluid is often possible.

Another exception to the above formulation is that of infection due to *P. pseudomallei*. This organism appears to be a free-living soil and water saprophyte in certain tropical areas, and it is capable of producing a broad spectrum of clinical illness in man and other mammals. Disease ranges from inapparent infection, to the pulmonary form of the disease, which is intermediate in severity, to the acute septicemic form of infection, which is highly lethal. With the recent military activity in Southeast Asia, this organism has become of more importance to physicians and health workers in the United States and Europe. The acute pulmonary form is the most common clinical manifestation of melioidosis. This may present as a mild bronchitis and bronchopneumonia or an overwhelming necrotizing pneumonia. A chronic suppurative form of the infection may be associated with pulmonary lesions many months to years after the patient has left the endemic area. Acute pulmonary infection is ordinarily characterized by an abrupt to subacute onset with anorexia, headache, and generalized myalgia. Fever and pleuritic or aching chest pain are common, as are cough and expectoration. The sputum may be blood-tinged. Chest films usually show upper lobe consolidation, frequently with cavities resembling those seen in tuberculosis. Nodular lesions and thin-walled cavitary lesions may also be seen. The leukocyte count is normal to moderately elevated.

Specific diagnosis rests on isolation of the organism from sputum or blood. *Pseudomonas pseudomallei* may be isolated on ordinary laboratory media in 48 to 72 hours. Other confirmatory laboratory data include a hemagglutination test, an agglutination test, and a complement fixation test. A fourfold or greater rise in titer is necessary for specific serologic diagnosis. A complement fixation titer of 1:8 or greater or hemagglutination titer of 1:160 or greater is highly suggestive of infection. Negative or low serologic titers do not exclude active disease.

Antibiotic therapy for organisms in this group is variable, and specific therapy should be tailored according to antimicrobial susceptibility testing. As a general rule, carbenicillin, colistimethate, gentamicin, and polymyxin B are effective agents for most isolates. In the case of *P. pseudomallei,* chloramphenicol, kanamycin, novobiocin, and tetracycline are of value. As with other pneumonias due to gram-negative bacilli, attention to supportive and surgical care is as important as the antibiotic therapy.

Haemophilus. The organisms in this category belong to the species *H. influenzae* as well as to related *H. parainfluenzae.* These are small, gram-negative pleomorphic coccobacilli which are found as normal inhabitants of the upper respiratory tract. Most illness in infants and children is due to capsular antigen type B, while most illness in adults is caused by the noncapsulated types.

Respiratory tract infections in infants and young children include acute epiglottitis, bronchiolitis, bronchitis, and bronchopneumonia. Acute epiglottitis has a characteristic abrupt onset with sore throat, fever, hoarseness, and a crouplike cough. Usually the illness progresses rapidly to the point of severe air hunger and respiratory stridor with intercostal and supraclavicular retraction. On examination the swollen, reddened epiglottis can be seen easily, and its appearance is quite characteristic. Complete respiratory obstruction is not uncommon. Epiglottitis may occur also with bronchiolitis, or the bronchiolitis syndrome may occur independently. Some have suggested a relationship to type A *H. influenzae,* although it is possible that this syndrome is viral in origin. Bronchitis usually occurs in a patient with underlying chronic bronchitis. One difficulty in interpretation of this syndrome is that the same organisms may be isolated from individuals with chronic obstructive pulmonary disease in whom no apparent acute infectious process is present. Therefore, the exact etiologic relationship of acute exacerbations of bronchitis in individuals with chronic obstructive pulmonary disease is not completely clear.

At times *H. influenzae,* usually type B, is associated with a bronchopneumonic illness—usually in children, occasionally in adults. In the latter case, the disease is frequently associated with some derangement of host defense mechanisms (diabetes mellitus, alcoholism, immunoglobulin deficiency state, and so on). The clinical features of the illness are not sufficiently characteristic to cause one to suspect this etiology. The best diagnostic clue is the appearance of characteristic small gram-negative coccobacillary forms in profusion on microscopical examination of the sputum.

Antimicrobial therapy of choice is ampicillin, with chloramphenicol being the agent of second choice. Other antimicrobial agents are more variable in their effectiveness.

Bacteroides and Related Anaerobes. The nonspore-forming gram-negative anaerobic bacilli, such as members of the *Bacteroides* and *Fusobacterium* genera, are common inhabitants of the upper respiratory tract (particularly in gingival sulci and tonsillar crypts) and the gastrointestinal tract. However, they are quite capable of producing many infectious illnesses in man. The lungs may be involved by aspiration of organisms from the mouth or pharynx, or the route of infection may be via septic thrombophlebitis and embolization from either the extremities or abdomen. Aspiration pneumonia and putrid lung abscess are almost universally mixed infections, sometimes containing several anaerobic organisms and frequently also containing aerobic organisms. In this type of infection the right upper lobe, because of its peculiar bronchial communication, is most frequently involved. Occasionally this type of pulmonary infection is associated with early pleural effusions or empyema. The characteristic history is that of a rather prolonged prodrome, with several days or weeks of fever, cough, weight loss, and extremely foul-smelling sputum, not infrequently occurring against the background of alcoholism. The syndrome due to infected pulmonary emboli usually follows abdominal or pelvic thrombophlebitis or surgery and is a more abrupt illness characterized by the development of metastatic lesions in the lungs.

The diagnosis is suggested primarily by the history and physical findings, particularly if there is foul-smelling sputum. Gram stain of sputum may show branching, filamentous, or otherwise pleomorphic organisms suggestive of anaerobes. Secretions for culture should be obtained in such a manner as to bypass the oropharynx. A definite diagnosis is also possible by isolating the organism by culture from pleural fluid, blood, or other exudates.

Most anaerobic gram-negative bacilli from the mouth are sensitive to penicillin and tetracyclines. On the basis of recent studies, however, clindamycin and chloramphenicol are emerging as the antimicrobial agents of choice in therapy of infections due to this class of organisms when the source is the abdomen or pelvis. Since antimicrobial susceptibility testing of anaerobic organisms is not a standardized, routine procedure, it should be attempted only by those individuals with sufficient competence to carry out the procedure and to interpret it appropriately.

Chlamydiae

This group of agents produces the diseases usually known as psittacosis, lymphogranuloma venereum, trachoma, and inclusion conjunctivitis. These organisms were previously considered to be large viruses, but in recent years they have come to be considered bacteria. Because the organisms are intracellular parasites, they do not grow on artificial media and require embryonated eggs or tissue cultures for detection. The most common agent in this group causing pulmonary infection is the psittacosis (ornithosis) agent. Human infection usually occurs as a consequence of exposure to pigeons, parakeets, parrots, or turkeys.

Psittacosis produces a severe pneumonia in man with mortality rates as high as 20%. After an incubation period of one to two weeks, the characteristic onset is sudden with chills, fever, anorexia, severe headache, malaise, and occasional other systemic symptoms. The fever is variable, and the course of the illness may be short (days) or prolonged (several weeks). The cough is usually nonproductive. Spleen and liver enlargement are sometimes present. Chest roentgenograms usually show the lung involvement to be more extensive than was expected on the basis of physical examination. The white blood cell count is usually normal, although occasionally low values are seen. Complications include severe anoxia and myocarditis. Fatal cases are usually associated with cyanosis. Diagnosis is based upon a history of contact with birds and by demonstrating a rising titer of complement fixing or agglutinating antibody. The organism can be cultured in embryonated eggs. The tetracyclines or chloramphenicol are agents of choice in antibiotic therapy.

Mycoplasma

Mycoplasma pneumoniae is the only mycoplasma known to cause human pneumonia, and the original syndrome of atypical pneumonia was ultimately found to be due to this organism (Eaton agent). *Mycoplasma hominis* is capable of producing pharyngitis. Pneumonia occurs in approximately 5 to 10% of patients found to be infected. The exact epidemiology is uncertain, but epidemic outbreaks occur particularly among military recruits and in young adult populations, although any age may be involved. Person-to-person spread is somewhat slow, with a two- or three-week interval being common. Clinical illness is also quite variable, ranging from relatively asymptomatic individuals to severe disease. Fever, malaise, weakness, and cough are the most common symptoms. Physical examination usually reveals only harsh breath sounds and an occasional wheeze. By contrast, chest roentgenograms may show localized to rather diffuse involvement that is more extensive than would have been expected on the basis of physical findings. Prolonged asthenia during convalescence is common.

The diagnosis rests upon clinical findings and the demonstration of rising titers of cold agglutinins and agglutinins to streptococcus MG. Specific mycoplasma complement fixation or agglutination tests are useful if available. In laboratories so prepared, the organism may be isolated either from pharyngeal washings or sputum.

It has been demonstrated that the illness can be shortened by administration of tetracycline or erythromycin. However, the response is not dramatic, and despite antibiotic therapy the organism can be recovered from throat cultures for many months. Specific vaccines are being investigated particularly for use in military recruit camps.

Rickettsiae

These pleomorphic rodlike structures are obligate intracellular parasites and are considered to be the smallest of the bacterial agents. Although pulmonary disease may be caused by many rickettsiae, *Coxiella burnetii* is the most common member of the group to produce pneumonia (Q fever). The natural reservoir of this organism is rodents, cattle, sheep, and goats, and it may be transmitted between these species by various ticks. The mode of transmission of *C. burnetii* to man is by inhalation of an infectious aerosol. Transmission to man via tick bite or human-to-human transmission has not been conclusively demonstrated. Individuals working in animal husbandry, dairies, abattoirs, and lambing pens are at greatest risk. The organism is somewhat resistant to physical and chemical agents and can survive long periods in dust.

The incubation period of the disease is from two to four weeks with the onset being abrupt and similar to many other influenzalike illnesses. Myalgia, headache, and retroorbital pain are rather characteristic. Some individuals have chest pain early in the course of illness, and others continue with this complaint throughout the course of disease. A dry cough is usually present. Unlike most rickettsial diseases, Q fever is not accompanied by a rash. Physical examination usually reveals a relative bradycardia, high fever, muscle tenderness, and occasionally neck stiffness. As with mycoplasma and chlamydia infections, the chest radiograph is considerably more remarkable than the physical examination. Pronounced changes may be present, ranging from bronchopneumonic infiltrates and areas of consolidation to diffuse miliary nodular infiltrates. Although individual patients may be quite seriously ill, the mortality rate is low.

The diagnosis of Q fever is quite difficult unless one has a high index of clinical suspicion. The illness is sufficiently similar to many other viral, bacterial, and fungal infections as to be nonspecific. The diagnosis is established either by isolating the organism in embryonated eggs or in animal inoculation or by use of the specific complement fixation test. A fourfold or greater rise in titer over a period of two weeks or more is necessary to establish the diagnosis. Unlike most other rickettsial diseases, the Weil-Felix reaction is negative. Because the organism is dangerous to laboratory workers and because the method of isolation from blood or respiratory secretions is extremely laborious, it is attempted only in a few reference laboratories.

Chloramphenicol or tetracyclines are indicated in the therapy of Q fever.

Actinomyces and Nocardia

Although these are often considered to be fungi, they are not taxonomically related to the true fungi. Both belong to the order Actinomycetales and the family Actinomycetaceae. *Actinomyces* species are anaerobic, while *Nocardia* species are aerobic. Nocardiae are relatively closely related to the Group 4 rapid-growing mycobacteria. Most pulmonary disease caused by nocardiae is due to *N. asteroides,* a weakly acid-fast branched mycelial organism that fragments into bacillary and coccoid forms. The organism is a saprophyte in soil, and infection is caused by inhalation. It has, on occasion, been found in sputum in otherwise healthy individuals, which suggests that the disease may at times be a self-limited primary pulmonary infection.

Clinical pulmonary nocardiosis varies from a mild to rather severe illness. It may be indistinguishable from certain forms of pulmonary tuberculosis or systemic fungal infections, on the one hand, and from acute bacterial pneumonia on the other. The course of infection is often punctuated by extrapulmonary manifestations, particularly abscesses in various sites of the body, including the brain. There are no particular physical or roentgenographic findings.

Diagnosis is based on culture of the organism from respiratory secretions. Microscopical examination of sputum may reveal mycelial forms or pus-containing sulfur granules. There are no serologic tests of value. Therapy is most satisfactory when sulfonamides are given for long periods of time (several weeks to several months). Cycloserine has been used successfully in a few patients.

Whereas nocardiae may be classified as exogenous organisms, actinomycetes are endogenous. *Actinomyces israelii* is the most common member of this group producing human disease. Its natural habitat is apparently the human oral cavity and gastrointestinal tract, and it grows under anaerobic conditions. Disease occurs as a result of implantation after trauma to oral tissues or after aspiration of oral contents.

There are classically three clinical forms of disease: (1) cervicofacial, (2) thoracic, and (3) abdominal. The thoracic form may begin as a pneumonic focus which may spread in a circumferential fashion and which characteristically crosses tissue planes and barriers, such as interlobar fissures or pleural boundaries, and may even involve ribs and chest wall tissues. Roentgenograms may reveal such spread and should alert one to the possibility of actinomycosis.

The diagnosis is made by demonstrating the typical sulfur granule in exudates or biopsy specimens and, rarely, in sputum. The granule contains clublike ends of hyphal structures arranged in a radial fashion around a dark-staining central mass of mycelial elements. The organism may be cultured from such material if it is handled in an anaerobic fashion. Expectorated sputum should not be cultured in this fashion because the organism appears normally in the mouth. There are no reliable serologic or skin tests available.

Antibiotic treatment of choice is penicillin G or ampicillin in moderately large doses for several months. Other antimicrobial agents, such as the tetracyclines, are less effective but may be used in the case of penicillin sensitivity. Cures have been reported following treatment with lincomycin and the cephalosporins. Surgical treatment is frequently necessary for drainage of pus and removal of necrotic tissues.

Fungi

A detailed description of the many pulmonary syndromes related to systemic and superficial fungi is beyond the scope of this chapter. The reader is referred to other available sources for such descriptions. Both acute self-limited and more progressive and chronic forms of pulmonary infection are frequently seen after inhalation of *Histoplasma capsulatum, Coccidioides immitis, Cryptococcus neoformans,* and *Blastomyces dermatitidis.* In addition, pulmonary infection due to *Sporotrichum schenckii* is occasionally seen.

Certain fungal agents are seen frequently as causing opportunistic infections in compromised hosts. These include various *Candida* species, *Mucor, Rhizopus,* and *Aspergillus* species. Pulmonary infections due to *Aspergillus* may be of three varieties—first, as a primary pulmonary infection; second, as a fungus ball (mycetoma) within a pulmonary cyst or cavity; and third, as a presumed allergic bronchopulmonary disorder. Other organisms rarely associated with pulmonary infections include *Torulopsis glabrata, Geotrichum candidum,* and *Paracoccidioides brasiliensis,* and there are others even more rare.

In recent years a number of thermophilic actinomycetes have been recognized as causes of hypersensitivity or allergic bronchopulmonary disorders. Most of these disorders are related to occupational exposure. The prototype of this disease is farmer's lung, in which inhalation of *Thermopolyspora polyspora* or *Micromonospora vulgaris* results in a progressive syndrome characterized by dyspnea, cough, and chest pain and tightness. The syndrome is presumed to be a hypersensitivity phenomenon because of the presence in the patient's serum of antibodies to these organisms. An ever-growing group of these disorders is being discovered, including maple bark disease, bagassosis, sequoiosis, and others. A similar syndrome has been described after exposure to such organisms present in central air conditioning and heating systems. Victims of these syndromes are relieved by removal from contact with the offending organisms.

Parasitic Infections

Pneumocystis carinii, which has become prominent in recent years, is classified loosely as a protozoan, although its exact taxonomy is indefinite. It is an oval or spheroidal parasite of 1 to 5 μ in diameter that occurs in a thin, cystlike structure. Many single parasites may occur within such cysts, which may be as large as 10 to 14 μ in diameter. The organism is frequently found in the lungs of healthy rodents and small domestic animals in whom no pathogenic relationship can be established. Normal rats become colonized in the lungs with this organism when treated with corticosteroids.

Most early reports of infection were from Europe in premature infants and young children compromised from other illnesses. In that context, it was seen as a cause of an interstitial pneumonia with plasma cell infiltrates. In the United States, infections due to *P. carinii* are seen most frequently in compromised hosts, both children and adults (e.g., in patients receiving steroids or immunosuppressive agents for malignant diseases or for organ transplantation, and in individuals with immunoglobulin deficiency states).

Clinical illness usually begins rather gradually with generalized symptoms such as weight loss, anorexia, malaise, and later the development of respiratory symptoms such as cough, dyspnea, and cyanosis.

Despite rather prominent symptoms in advanced disease, physical findings in the chest are remarkable for their paucity or absence. This is further contrasted by the finding on the chest film of rather marked infiltrates extending from the hilar regions toward the periphery in a butterfly fashion. Later the roentgenographic findings include dense infiltrates with surrounding hyperinflation or occasional pneumothorax. Laboratory findings are not otherwise remarkable except as they reflect the underlying disease process. Although most cases terminate in death, the significance of this fact is uncertain because of the serious underlying disease which is almost invariably present.

Diagnosis is based on morphologic demonstration of the organism in specimens obtained usually by lung biopsy or transthoracic aspiration. These are best seen on periodic acid–Schiff or methenamine silver stains. It is unusual to see these organisms on specimens of respiratory secretions. The organism has never been cultivated on artificial media, and there are no serologic diagnostic methods available at present.

Many cases have been treated successfully with pentamidine isethionate, which can be obtained only by special request from the Center for Disease Control in Atlanta. There are scattered reports of seemingly successful therapy using sulfonamide plus either pyrimethamine or trimethoprim.

Viruses

It is beyond the purview of this chapter to examine in detail the viruses capable of causing respiratory disease. Table 4-1 will serve as a guide to the reader in establishing etiologic relationships of viruses and respiratory syndromes. Viruses are known to be capable of producing many clinical syndromes, such as coryza (the common cold), pharyngitis, laryngitis, croup, tracheobronchitis, bronchiolitis, pleurodynia, and almost any type of pneumonia. Viruses most commonly linked with pneumonic illnesses include influenza and parainfluenza, adenoviruses, varicella, measles, and cytomegalovirus. The last has been found most frequently in patients with malignant diseases or organ transplants and in whom immunosuppressive drugs have been used.

There is suggestive evidence that prompt treatment with amantadine in patients with influenza may be beneficial. This agent has also been shown to be of prophylactic benefit in protecting individuals after exposure to influenza A. There also are several reports of efficacy of cytosine arabinoside in varicella-zoster infection. It is likely that antiviral chemotherapy will become a practical reality within the next decade.

TABLE 4-1 / Viruses and Acute Respiratory Diseases

		Clinical Syndromes								
Viruses	Major Types	Coryza	Gingivo-stomatitis	Pharyn-gitis	Laryn-gitis	Croup	Tracheo-bronchitis	Bronchi-olitis	Pleuro-dynia	Pneumonia
Adenoviruses	1–7, 14, 15, 21	. . .	. . .	+	. . .	. . .	. . .	. . .	. . .	+
Herpes viruses										
Herpes virus hominis (simplex)		. . .	+	. . .	. . .	. . .	. . .	. . .	. . .	. . .
Varicella-zoster		. . .	. . .	. . .	. . .	. . .	+	. . .	. . .	+
Cytomegalovirus		. . .	. . .	. . .	. . .	. . .	. . .	. . .	. . .	+
Myxoviruses										
Influenza	A, A_1, A_2, B	. . .	. . .	. . .	. . .	. . .	+	. . .	. . .	+
Parainfluenza	1, 2, 3	+	. . .	+	+	+	+	. . .	. . .	+
Measles (rubeola)		+	. . .	. . .	. . .	. . .	+	. . .	. . .	+
Picornaviruses										
Coxsackie virus										
Group A	2–10, 21	. . .	. . .	+	. . .	. . .	. . .	. . .	. . .	. . .
Group B	1–6	. . .	. . .	. . .	. . .	. . .	. . .	. . .	+	. . .
REO viruses		+	. . .	. . .	. . .	. . .	. . .	. . .	. . .	. . .
Rhinoviruses		+	. . .	. . .	. . .	. . .	+ (?)	+ (?)	. . .	. . .
Others										
Infectious mono-nucleosis		. . .	. . .	+	. . .	. . .	. . .	. . .	. . .	. . .
Respiratory syncytial virus		+	. . .	. . .	. . .	. . .	. . .	+	. . .	+ (?)

REFERENCES

Anderson, J. P., and Bridgwater, F. A. J. Ornithosis in a chest clinic practice. *Brit. J. Dis. Chest* 62:155, 1968.

Austrian, R., and Gold, J. Pneumococcal bacteremia with especial reference to bacteremic pneumococcal pneumonia. *Ann. Intern. Med.* 60:759, 1964.

Bandt, P. D., Blank, N., and Castellino, R. A. Needle diagnosis of pneumonitis: Value in high-risk patients. *J.A.M.A.* 220:1578, 1972.

Barnett, J. A., Gilbert, D. N., Hyland, R. N., Luby, J. P., Newberry, W. M., Sanford, J. P., Shropshire, S., Smith, J. W., and Southern, P. M., Jr. *Guide to Antimicrobial Therapy: 1971.* Dallas: Sanford, 1971.

Barnett, T. B., and Herring, C. L. Lung abscess: Initial and late results of medical therapy. *Arch. Intern. Med.* (Chicago) 127:217, 1971.

Barrett-Connor, E. The nonvalue of sputum culture in the diagnosis of pneumococcal pneumonia. *Amer. Rev. Resp. Dis.* 103:845, 1971.

Bartlett, J. G., and Finegold, S. M. Clinical features and diagnosis of anaerobic pleuropulmonary infections. *Antimicrob. Agents Chemother.* 10:78, 1970.

Baum, G. L., Feldman, H. A., Lepper, M. H., Sanford, J. P., Wehrle, P. F., and Green, R. A. Definitions and classifications of infectious reactions of the lung. *Amer. Rev. Resp. Dis.* 101:1, 1970.

Chanock, R. *Mycoplasma* infections of man. *New Eng. J. Med.* 273:1197, 273:1257, 1965.

Cohen, H. I., Merigan, T. C., Kosek, J. C., and Eldridge, F. Sequoiosis: Granulomatous pneumonitis associated with sawdust inhalation. *Amer. J. Med.* 43:785, 1967.

Dailey, R. H., and Benner, E. J. Necrotizing pneumonitis due to the pseudomonad "eugonic oxidizer—Group I." *New Eng. J. Med.* 279:361, 1968.

DeVita, V. T., Emmer, M., Levine, A., Jacobs, B., and Berard, C. *Pneumocystis carinii* pneumonia. *New Eng. J. Med.* 280:287, 1969.

Dudding, B. A., Wagner, S. G., Zeller, J. A., Gmelich, J. T., French, G. R., and Top, F. H., Jr. Fatal pneumonia associated with adenovirus type 7 in three military trainees. *New Eng. J. Med.* 286:1289, 1972.

Edmondson, E. B., and Sanford, J. P. The *Klebsiella-Enterobacter* (*Aerobacter*)*-Serratia* group: A clinical and bacteriological evaluation. *Medicine* 46:323, 1967.

Fennessy, J. J. Bronchial brushing and transbronchial forceps biopsy in the diagnosis of pulmonary lesions. *Dis. Chest* 53:377, 1962.

Fetzer, A. E., Werner, A. S., and Hagstrom, J. W. C. Pathologic features of pseudomonal pneumonia. *Amer. Rev. Resp. Dis.* 96:1121, 1967.

Fink, J. N., Banaszak, E. F., Thiede, W. H., and Barboriak, J. J. Interstitial pneumonitis due to hypersensitivity to an organism contaminating a heating system. *Ann. Intern. Med.* 74:80, 1971.

Finland, M., Peterson, O. L., and Strauss, E. Staphylococcic pneumonia occurring during an epidemic of influenza. *Arch. Intern. Med.* 70:185, 1942.

Goldstein, E., Daly, A. K., and Seamans, S. *Haemophilus influenzae* as a cause of adult pneumonia. *Ann. Intern. Med.* 66:35, 1967.

Goodell, B., Jacobs, J. B., Powell, R. D., and DeVita, V. T. *Pneumocystis carinii:* The spectrum of diffuse interstitial pneumonia in patients with neoplastic diseases. *Ann. Intern. Med.* 72:337, 1970.

Hahn, H. D., and Beaty, H. N. Transtracheal aspiration in the evaluation of patients with pneumonia. *Ann. Intern. Med.* 72:183, 1970.

Hirschman, S. Z., Meyers, B. R., and Millian, S. J. The diagnostic microbiology of lung biopsy: Correlation with viral serology. *Mt. Sinai J. Med. N.Y.* 28:273, 1971.

Howe, C., Sampath, A., and Spotnitz, M. The pseudomallei group: A review. *J. Infect. Dis.* 124:598, 1971.

James, A. E., Dixon, G. D., and Johnson, H. F. Melioidosis: Correlation of radiologic and pathologic findings. *Radiology* 89:230, 1967.

Johanson, W. G., Pierce, A. K., and Sanford, J. P. Changing pharyngeal bacterial flora of hospitalized patients: Emergence of gram-negative bacilli. *New Eng. J. Med.* 281:1137, 1969.

Johnson, J. E., III, and Kadull, P. J. Laboratory-acquired Q fever: A report of fifty cases. *Amer. J. Med.* 41:391, 1966.

Kilbourn, J. P., Campbell, R. A., Grach, J. L., and Willis, M. D. Quantitative bacteriology of sputum. *Amer. Rev. Resp. Dis.* 98:810, 1968.

Krumholz, R. A., Manfredi, F., and Weg, J. G. Needle biopsy of the lung: Report of its use in 112 patients and review of the literature. *Ann. Intern. Med.* 65:293, 1966.

Laurenzi, G. A., Potter, R. T., and Kass, E. H. Bacteriologic flora of the lower respiratory tract. *New Eng. J. Med.* 265:1273, 1961.

Louria, D. B., Hensle, T., and Rose, J. The major medical complications of heroin addiction. *Ann. Intern. Med.* 67:1, 1967.

Manfredi, F., Daly, W. J., and Behnke, R. H. Clinical observations of acute Friedlander pneumonia. *Ann. Intern. Med.* 58:642, 1963.

Mays, B. B., Thomas, G. D., Leonard, J. S., Jr., Southern, P. M., Jr., Pierce, A. K., and Sanford, J. P. Gram-negative bacillary necrotizing pneumonia: A bacteriologic and histopathologic correlation. *J. Infect. Dis.* 120:687, 1969.

Peabody, J. W., Jr., and Seabury, J. H. Actinomycosis and nocardiosis. *J. Chronic Dis.* 5:374, 1957.

Peabody, J. W., Jr., and Seabury, J. H. Actinomycosis and nocardiosis: A review of basic differences in therapy. *Amer. J. Med.* 28:99, 1960.

Pecora, D. V., and Kohl, M. Transtracheal aspiration in the diagnosis of acute lower respiratory tract infection. *Amer. Rev. Resp. Dis.* 86:755, 1962.

Pierce, A. K., Edmondson, E. B., McGee, G., Ketchersid, J., Loudon, R. G., and Sanford, J. P. An analysis of factors predisposing to gram-negative bacillary necrotizing pneumonia. *Amer. Rev. Resp. Dis.* 94:309, 1966.

Rahal, J. J., Jr., Meade, R. H., III, Bump, C. M., and Reinauer, A. J. Upper respiratory tract carriage of gram-negative enteric bacilli by hospital personnel. *J.A.M.A.* 214:754, 1970.

Scerbo, J., Keltz, H., and Stone, D. J. A prospective study of closed pleural biopsies. *J.A.M.A.* 218:377, 1971.

Shames, J. M., George, R. B., Holliday, W. B., Rasch, J. R., and Mogabgab, W. J. Comparisons of antibiotics in the treatment of mycoplasmal pneumonia. *Arch. Intern. Med.* 125:680, 1970.

Slavin, R. G. Allergic bronchopulmonary aspergillosis—a North American rarity: Clinical and immunologic characteristics. *Amer. J. Med.* 47:306, 1969.

Spencer, C. D., and Beaty, H. N. Complications of transtracheal aspiration. *New Eng. J. Med.* 286:304, 1972.

Tillotson, J. R., and Finland, M. Bacterial colonization and clinical superinfection of the respiratory tract complicating antibiotic treatment of pneumonia. *J. Infect. Dis.* 119:597, 1969.

Tillotson, J. R., and Lerner, A. M. Pneumonias caused by gram negative bacilli. *Medicine* 45:65, 1966.

Tillotson, J. R., and Lerner, A. M. *Bacteroides* pneumonias: Characteristics of cases with empyema. *Ann. Intern. Med.* 68:308, 1968.

Tillotson, J. R., and Lerner, A. M. Characteristics of nonbacteremic pseudomonas pneumonia. *Ann. Intern. Med.* 68:295, 1968.

5 / BACTERIAL MENINGITIS

J. Joseph Marr

There are few instances in which the introduction of modern chemotherapy has produced such gratifying results as it has in the treatment of bacterial meningitis. Prior to the advent of antibiotics, pyogenic meningitis was almost uniformly fatal, and in survivors residual damage to the nervous system was frequently severe. However, despite effective antibiotics and improvements in the management of shock, bacterial meningitis still remains a life-threatening problem which taxes the abilities of the most adept clinician. In the past fifteen years there has been no significant change in the death rate due to this disease. This is especially true with regard to the newborn; neonates are the major contributors to this persistent morbidity and mortality.

NEONATAL MENINGITIS

Meningitis is more common in the first month of life than in any succeeding month. The results of the National Collaborative Perinatal Research Study indicated that 25 cases of neonatal meningitis were identified among 54,535 live births, an incidence of 0.46 per 1,000. In virtually all reported series of meningitis in this age group, including those from the larger medical centers, mortality has ranged from 50 to 90% and at present is about 65% on the average. Another aspect of concern is that there are significant permanent sequelae in a large number of survivors of neonatal meningitis.

Probable factors for this high rate of death and incidence of sequelae include the following: the symptoms and signs of meningitis in the neonatal period are sufficiently nonspecific and undramatic to allow a relatively large number of cases to go unrecognized; the most frequent causative organisms are gram-negative enteric bacilli, many of which are resistant to antibiotics and refractory to treatment. The predilection to infection by gram-negative organisms which rarely cause meningitis in older children may also reflect the effect of maternal parapartum infections or exposure to these organisms through humidification apparatus, resuscitation equipment, or articles used in daily care in the nursery. Neonates who develop meningitis have often required one or all of these items of equipment. Obstetrical abnormalities late in pregnancy occur frequently in mothers of infants who develop meningitis during the first weeks of life. These include premature births, traumatic delivery, premature rupture of the membranes, prolonged labor, and maternal infection. The age of onset of meningitis is significantly earlier in infants born of women with perinatal obstetrical complications, which suggests that infection often occurs either in utero or during delivery. Premature birth is the most common abnormality.

There are also several contributing neonatal factors. Meningitis results as a sequela to sepsis or from direct extension of an infection from other organs. A variety of portals of entry have been encountered in neonatal meningitis and include the gastrointestinal, respiratory, and urinary tracts, the middle ear, the skin, and the umbilicus. The neonate with infection in any of these organs, systems, or sites has an increased risk of developing meningitis.

In general, the younger and smaller the infant, the more nonspecific are the clinical symptoms and signs. Fever, for example, is frequently absent in neonates with serious infections. Many infants in the first days of life have a rectal temperature of 36°C., so a rise in temperature during this time may be overlooked because of this developmental feature. Leukocytosis may or may not be present. Neurologic manifestations appear relatively late in the course of illness, if at all. Changes in the tension of the anterior fontanelle are present in less than 40% of infants and nuchal rigidity in fewer than 10%. Thus, diagnosis must rest on a high index of suspicion and a liberal and early use of blood cultures and examination of the cerebrospinal fluid. In a review of the literature [1] of neonatal meningitis, 72% of 146 blood cultures were positive and yielded the same organism as that recovered from the spinal fluid. Blood cultures should be obtained from peripheral veins, since those obtained from catheterized umbilical vessels may yield falsely positive results. The pour-plate technique is useful in distinguishing skin or laboratory contamination of cultures.

A wide variety of bacteria may cause neonatal meningitis. However, the common etiologic agents of purulent meningitis of older infants, children, and adults are rarely seen in neonatal meningitis (see Table 5-1). Fosson and Fine [1] have shown that the causative organisms in 478 patients with neonatal meningitis were gram-negative enteric bacteria in 295 (62%) of the cases. *Escherichia coli* was the most common causative organism, accounting for 195 cases. Other genera of gram-negative bacteria, in order of frequency, were *Paracolobactrum, Proteus, Pseudomonas, Salmonella,* and *Klebsiella-Enterobacter.* The streptococcus was the second most frequent organism, accounting for 45 cases (9.6%); group B streptococci were the most frequent offenders. Twenty-six cases were due to staphylococci and 27 to pneumococci.

There is an intimate relationship between the type of causative organism and the pathogenesis of meningitis in the neonate. Neonates with meningitis due to gram-negative bacteria are likely to have a history of perinatal abnormalities, to be of low birth weight, and to have an early onset of disease. Those with infections due to streptococci and staphylococci usually have a later onset and an absence of perinatal abnormalities, which suggests that such infections were contracted postnatally by other routes. The role of skin infection, including omphalitis or dermal sinus infection, is especially important [2].

There are differences in the immunologic capabilities of the developing individual and the older child or adult which may play a role in the increased susceptibility of the neonate to infection. The prematurely born infant is deprived of his full supply of passively transferred antibody to a degree that parallels his low birth weight, and the newborn infant has been shown to have a lack of serum bactericidins against gram-negative bacteria. These antibodies against the somatic bacterial antigens are in the immunoglobulin M (IgM) fraction which is not passed transplacentally from mother to fetus. This relative paucity of IgM in the normal newborn as compared with the adult has been thought to be partially responsible for the susceptibility of neonates to gram-negative bacterial infections.

Early diagnosis is probably the single most important factor in reducing morbidity and mortality in neonatal meningitis. For example, the mortality rates in several series of patients from large medical centers varies from 60% to 75%, and of 236 patients reported in twelve groups of patients throughout the world who were treated with penicillin and an antibiotic active against gram-negative organisms, 157 (66%) died. Optimal antibody therapy is not enough; it must be allied with an early diagnosis. In 101 neonates who died from meningitis, the mean duration before the initiation of therapy was 5.3 days. In 19 severely damaged infants it was 5.4 days, whereas in 32 survivors without sequelae, only 2 days elapsed before antimicrobial therapy was initiated.

MENINGITIS IN CHILDREN AND ADULTS

The symptoms of acute bacterial meningitis in adults are well known. Most patients have fever, headache, irritability, lethargy or confusion, and vomiting. Nuchal rigidity is usually present. The onset may be insidious or rapidly progressive over a period of several hours; if the latter, mortality is generally higher. Disease due to the meningococcus generally evolves rapidly, whereas that seen in childhood due to *Haemophilus influenzae* is somewhat slower. About half of the patients with meningococcal meningitis will have petechiae or purpuric skin lesions. Although these lesions are helpful in diagnosis, similar lesions, together with cerebrospinal fluid pleocytosis, are seen in conditions other than meningococcal disease. Examples include aseptic meningitis due to type 9 ECHO virus, acute bacterial endocarditis, and, occasionally, meningitis due to bacteria other than the meningococcus.

Older infants and children have more prominent symptomatology than the neonate. Fever, headache, vomiting, and the customary signs of meningeal irritation are the presenting complaints. Cranial bruits have recently been described as a clinical sign in diagnosis of meningitis in these patients [3]. The bruit is transitory and disappears after therapy. About two-thirds of children with meningococcal disease will have an exanthem. Although skin lesions are petechial when fully developed, a macular rash may appear initially. Erythema nodosum has also been observed. Petechial skin lesions are seen in children with meningococcemia and are less common in meningitis due to other organisms.

Joint involvement may be seen in about 5% of patients with meningococcal disease. Some patients, especially those with fulminant disease, may have arthritis of several joints due to direct bacterial seeding of the synovia. An apparent hypersensitivity arthritis with onset late in the first week of the illness may pose a diagnostic dilemma. Joint pain with a sterile effusion is characteristic. This form of arthritis does not require special treatment and generally subsides within a week or two; sequelae are unknown. Septicemia with other organisms produces an arthritis different from that of the meningococcus. A purulent arthritis with active multiplication of bacteria in the joint spaces is seen; prompt drainage (either open or closed) is necessary to prevent joint destruction and ankylosis.

About 10% of patients with acute bacterial meningitis will have established or impending shock when first seen. Shock may be unrecognized in young infants but should be suspected in those with subnormal temperatures.

THEORIES OF PATHOGENESIS AND THEIR IMPLICATIONS FOR PROGNOSIS

The pathogenesis of meningitis may be elucidated by contrasting the disease as produced by the meningococcus with that caused by the pneumococcus. The former serves as the prototype of an infection which begins at a locus distant from the meninges, produces a bacteremia, and ultimately results in central nervous system (CNS) disease. Pneumococcal meningitis, by contrast, frequently begins as local cranial disease (otitis, sinusitis) and may be used as a model of bacterial invasion of the CNS from an adjacent focus. In the latter instance, bacteremia follows the meningitis and is secondary to it. Thus, bacteremia differs in its import in pneumococcal as opposed to meningococcal meningitis. Dowling's view that the presence or absence of bacteremia in meningococcal meningitis is of little value in predicting the outcome is now generally held [4], since most, if not all, cases of meningococcal meningitis result from an antecedent meningococcemia. In distinction, pneumococcal meningitis may result either from bacteremia or direct extension of infection from a cephalic focus. Bacteremia is of grave prognostic import in pneumococcal meningitis.

Meningococcal meningitis and septicemia are relatively rare when considered relative to the numbers of nasopharyngeal carriers; the carrier state reflects the true prevalence of the organism in our population. Moreover, since it is accompanied by an antibody response [5, 6], the carrier state is considered to be a true infection. Observations in military recruits have suggested a close association of respiratory disease and meningococcal infection. One study has indicated, however, that the relationship is apparently not one of cause and effect [7]. In this investigation significant reduction in viral respiratory disease in a military population followed the use of an adenovirus vaccine, yet meningococcal carrier rates were virtually identical to those of a corresponding nonimmunized group. Interestingly, the carrier rates of both groups increased progressively from an initial 33% to over 80% at the sixth week of basic training, yet no case of meningococcal meningitis occurred in over 950 individuals studied. The majority of meningococcal infections of the nasopharynx occurred either before the onset of, or in the absence of, viral proliferation in the upper respiratory tract. This suggests that viral respiratory disease is not a significant factor in the dissemination of meningococcal disease among recruits and is unlikely to be the cause of CNS invasion following the nasopharyngeal acquisition of the meningococcus.

Pneumococcal meningitis has a varied provenance. In some patients meningitis complicates pneumococcal pneumonia and bacteremia; in others, paranasal sinus or middle ear infection may extend directly to the upper respiratory tract and thence to the meninges, without an intervening bacteremia. There are potentially four groups of patients with pneumococcal meningitis: those with a cephalic portal of entry, with or without bacteremia, and those with a pulmonary portal of entry, with or without bacteremia. Since bacteremia seldom appears in association with sinusitis or otitis alone [8], the bacteremia seen in pneumococcal meningitis from sinus or ear disease most likely follows the meningeal invasion. One might thus expect that individuals with pneumococcal meningitis plus bacteremia would not fare as well as persons with meningitis alone. This expectation was proved correct in a study reported by Austrian [8]. Among 13 persons with otitis or sinusitis and meningitis, but without bacteremia, no fatalities occurred; in 27 persons with otitis or sinusitis and meningitis with bacteremia, there were 17 deaths—a fatality rate of 63%. Similarly, in 24 cases of pneumonia with bacteremia the fatality rate was 83%, whereas in pneumonia without bacteremia the mortality rate was about 10%.

From these observations it could be inferred that adequate doses of pneumococcidal drugs, such as penicillin, would control the meningeal and neural infection; this is correct. The toxemia that accompanies bacteremia at the time treatment is begun is, however, relatively uninfluenced by antimicrobial therapy and is a factor leading to the death of the bacteremic patient. The high mortality associated with bacteremia also reflects the fact that the host defense mechanisms are severely compromised by the infection or bacteremia would not have occurred. In meningococcal meningitis, the presence or absence of bacteremia at the time of hospitalization has little effect on the outcome [9].

Austrian's work [8] yields another item of interest. In his study of pneumococcal pneumonia and meningitis there were differences in the incidence of bacteremia: 28% in pneumonia and 68% in meningitis. Several studies of experimental pneumococcal meningitis and experimental pneumococcal pneumonia have indicated that the membranes interposed between the subarachnoid space and the cerebral venous circulation are distinctly less effective than the cellular and anatomic barriers between the pulmonary lymphatics and the thoracic duct and subclavian vein. Isotope-labeled erythrocytes placed in the subarachnoid space produce no radioactivity in the cervical lymph nodes, although labeled cells appear in the circulation. Similar results have been found using dye-labeled protein. Of more interest are the studies by Welch and Pollay [10], in which the excised dural sinuses of monkeys were perfused at physiologic pressures. These experiments demonstrated that fluid passed only in one direction, into the sagittal sinus. At comparable pressures yeast cells and erythrocytes were shown to pass in the same direction. It appears that a ready pathway exists for the passage of bacteria from the subarachnoid space to the cerebral venous circulation when the cerebrospinal fluid pressure is elevated. Studies by Austrian [8] have shown that the average cerebrospinal fluid pressure of patients with meningitis of cephalic origin plus bacteremia was about 100 mm. H_2O higher than that of their counterparts without bacteremia.

SYSTEMIC EFFECTS OF ENDOTOXIN IN THE CENTRAL NERVOUS SYSTEM

Several lines of evidence suggest that gram-negative endotoxin may act on the CNS to produce systemic effects [11, 12]. Penner and Bernheim [11] have demonstrated that the ulcerative gastrointestinal tract lesions of systemic canine endotoxemia are also demonstrable after the introduction of *Shigella* endotoxin into the third ventricle in doses which are completely innocuous when given systemically. These changes can be prevented by prior splanchnic denervation [13]. There is additional evidence that ganglionic blocking drugs and α-adrenergic blockade may prevent the physiologic effects of endotoxin [14]. Taken collectively, the above implicate the autonomic nervous system in the pathogenesis of endotoxin shock. Kass and his co-workers have observed that in rats, *E. coli* endotoxin is lethal at lower doses when given by intracarotid injection than by intravenous injection. This phenomenon can be greatly modified by ablation of the posterior hypothalamus [15]. It is not clear whether sympathetic activity is induced by endotoxin directly or is a reflex event initiated in another manner.

The systemic pathology seen in meningitis [16, 17] may also be induced by the action of bacterial products on particular areas of the CNS in concentrations that are innocuous when given systemically. Sterile meningococcal endotoxin placed within the ventricular system of dogs produces a marked systemic reaction [18]: 4 mg. per kilogram of body weight of meningococcal endotoxin was lethal for 7 of 8 dogs when injected into the third ventricle, whereas the same amount of endotoxin given intravenously to 7 dogs was not lethal. An additional 7 animals injected with saline into the third ventricle suffered no adverse effects. All animals given intraventricular endotoxin were hyperthermic and appeared extremely ill, with nearly all exhibiting vomiting, anorexia, and variable levels of consciousness. These animals demonstrated hyperemia within the walls of the injected ventricle and an acute ependymitis up to six cells in depth of all ventricles, being most marked in the third. There were no discernible hypothalamic lesions.

The most striking finding at autopsy in these animals was massive pulmonary edema. The pleural surfaces were congested, and on sectioning blood and edema fluid were easily seen. Subendocardial hemorrhage was present in both ventricles, and the mitral valve was swollen and hemorrhagic. There were similar changes in the tricuspid valve, although the pulmonic and aortic valves appeared normal. No myocardial necrosis or zonal lesions could be found. Liver congestion was evident at gross examination, although hepatic cellular necrosis was not found. The spleen was normal. The kidneys demonstrated mild hyperemia at the corticomedullary junction. Glomeruli were moderately congested without thrombosis or infarction on microscopical examination. The gross appearance of the adrenal glands was normal, but sectioning revealed congestion. Moderate to marked hemorrhage was present at the junction of the adrenal medulla and cortex in 3 of 7 animals, but the medulla itself was normal and no vascular lesions were demonstrable. Gross examination of the gastrointestinal mucosa revealed hyperemia, especially marked in the prepyloric region, the duodenum, and the proximal colon. Most of the intestine was normal to microscopical examination save for a few areas of local vascular congestion which did not involve the entire bowel circumference. There were no lesions noted in the skin. Postmortem examination revealed no CNS pathology in dogs receiving either intravenous endotoxin or intraventricular saline.

A more recent attempt to define the role of the central nervous system in septic shock demonstrated that the intravenous LD_{80} dose of endotoxin could be reduced by one-half if the endotoxin was placed intracisternally [19]. Instilling the endotoxin within the ventricle decreased the LD_{80} to one-fifth that of the intravenous route. The LD_{80} of endotoxin in the thoracic subarachnoid space was not different from that in intravenous injection. Animals injected with saline were unharmed.

The pathologic changes of systemic endotoxemia have been described by a number of investigators [20] and are slightly different from those mentioned above. Most studies, however, have been incidental to physiologic investigations and have been somewhat incomplete. The lesions within the gastrointestinal tract usually begin at the pylorus and extend for a variable distance beyond the ligament of Treitz. The mucosa is hyperemic with a nonuniform distribution and with minute, dark red petechial lesions interspersed among areas which are variously congested. Microscopically the earliest changes are congestion and distention of the capillaries in the tips of the villi, with submucosal edema and sloughing of the villi. In animals dying of systemic endotoxin shock, these changes are present throughout the entire gastrointestinal tract. The same changes can be elicited by hemorrhagic shock or by the infusion of epinephrine [13, 21].

The extent of the pathologic change achieved by the lethal CNS injection of endotoxin resembles most closely the early lesions found in systemic endotoxemia. The fact that such lesions can be induced by hemorrhage or the infusion of epinephrine and can be prevented in some circumstances by splanchnic denervation and ganglionic blocking agents suggests that in the dog they are the result of a nonspecific sympathetic discharge. The pathologic changes found in the heart and lungs, liver, adrenal glands, and kidneys in both intravenous and CNS endotoxin shock are similar and consist primarily of severe congestion.

The pathologic changes which follow injection of a small amount of endotoxin in the CNS differ in degree rather than in kind from those changes found in animals with severe endotoxemia. Thus, it is highly likely that the systemic changes seen during intracranial infections may depend to some extent on the presence of intracranial endotoxin and its effects on those higher centers which can be reached by diffusion from the ventricular system.

In autopsy series of meningococcal meningitis with meningococcemia, systemic pathologic changes generally dominate those found in the CNS [16, 17]. Nevertheless, there are many such cases in which the septicemia has not been documented. The usual explanation given for the presence of systemic pathology in the absence of a demonstrable septicemia is the fastidious growth requirements of the organisms. However, from the experiments cited above and from other investigations of CNS contributions to the total picture of septic shock, it is becoming evident that endotoxin of gram-negative organisms infecting the CNS can cause many systemic effects. The ability of the endotoxin to cause systemic pathologic lesions and death depends to some degree on the proximity of the endotoxin to higher nervous centers.

These experimental results coincide rather well with many of the pathologic changes found in patients dying with meningococcal meningitis. Both central and peripheral actions of the endotoxin are doubtless operative in meningococcal infections, but the fact that the illness is often refractory to antibiotic therapy despite sterilization of both blood and spinal fluid suggests that the central effects of endotoxin may be critical to survival. Future studies in this area should yield valuable new clinical and investigative concepts.

DIAGNOSIS

The single most important factor in prognosis is the period of time between diagnosis and onset of therapy. In its early stages meningitis may be easily misdiagnosed as a viral-like illness when there is only modest fever, headache, and minimal stiffness of the neck. It is often impossible to distinguish early meningitis from a viral illness without performing a lumbar puncture, and this must be done whenever the diagnosis is considered. The decision regarding lumbar puncture may be based on the presence or absence of signs of meningeal irritation; a sensitive test is to ask the patient to place his head between his knees while sitting in bed. When a diagnosis is in doubt, it is not advisable to await clear-cut signs of meningeal irritation before performing a lumbar puncture. The experimental results previously described should serve as a stimulus to the clinician, since the presence of CNS endotoxin or secondary bacteremia is associated with a higher mortality.

Mental symptoms may predominate in any type of meningitis, but these are more prevalent in tuberculosis and syphilitic or other spirochetal infections. Confusion or delirium may be erroneously ascribed to alcoholism, senility, drugs, diabetes, or a stroke. Consideration of other neurologic disorders may frequently delay the proper diagnosis. The onset of meningococcal meningitis may be so sudden and dramatic as to suggest a subarachnoid hemorrhage or a cerebrovascular accident. Head trauma with skull fracture may provide ingress to bacteria from the nose, sinuses, or ears; on these occasions the signs of meningitis may be ascribed to blood in the subarachnoid space. Brain abscess with secondary meningitis may be misinterpreted as a brain tumor with associated hemorrhage. Other infections, when present, may provide a ready explanation for the fever and headache and may delay the diagnosis of a coincidental meningitis. This is especially true when frontal sinusitis or otitis exists with fever and headache.

Pneumonia or septicemia with fever, headache, and delirium may also mask meningitis. Patients such as these should be closely followed and a lumbar puncture performed at the earliest indication. It is difficult to exclude an encephalitis, since most forms of meningitis are associated with a superficial cerebritis and since encephalitis is almost always accompanied by some degree of meningeal irritation. In this clinical situation meningitis should be considered first since most forms are amenable to specific antibiotic therapy, whereas most forms of encephalitis have no specific therapy. Encephalitis is a diagnosis of exclusion.

Laboratory Tests

At the time spinal fluid is obtained, two blood specimens for culture should be collected as well. The presence of papilledema on physical examination should not preclude the performance of lumbar puncture. Difficulty in obtaining fluid should alert the physician to the possibility of an epidural abscess or other obstruction. In bacterial meningitis organisms are seen on the spun sediment of the spinal fluid about two-thirds of the time.

Because of the fastidiousness of meningococci, warm chocolate agar (37°C.) should be inoculated and placed in a candle jar directly at the bedside. The temperature of the agar is important, since these organisms will not grow at temperatures much below 34°C. The agar may be brought to proper temperature by placing it under a bedside lamp. Blood, nasal swabs, and aspirates of skin lesions should be handled similarly, and cultures should be incubated both aerobically and anaerobically.

If a differential count shows mononuclear cells, acid-fast stains and India ink preparations should be examined. When a malignancy is suspected, a coverglass smear of the spun sediment may be prepared with a small amount of serum or albumin added in order to enable the cells to stick to the coverglass. If no organisms are demonstrated on the stained smear, repeat smears may be made aseptically from the cerebrospinal fluid after 6 to 8 hours of incubation. The concentration of glucose in the cerebrospinal fluid should be determined immediately and the concentration of glucose in the blood measured at the same time. If viral meningitis is a possibility, specimens of cerebrospinal fluid and serum should be frozen for subsequent study.

ETIOLOGY AND THERAPY

The most common pathogens found in bacterial meningitis are listed in Table 5-1. Meningitis in the newborn infant poses special problems in management, since the organisms recovered from these patients are quite different from those in older individuals. These enterobacteria are unusual in older children and adults. The most common organism found in infants is *H. influenzae*, type B, a common inhabitant of the nasopharynx in children. Most disease appears to occur either spontaneously or following a mild respiratory infection, although episodes apparently secondary to acute otitis media, pneumonia, or cellulitis are seen. From age 5 to 15 the meningococcus predominates. In adults the pneumococcus and meningococcus are almost equal in their frequency, although in most reported series of cases the pneumococcus is seen with slightly greater frequency.

Knowledge of the most probable pathogen found in each age group is of importance when the findings in the cerebrospinal fluid indicate that the infecting agent is bacterial but no organisms are recognized on a smear of the sediment. At these times therapy is directed against the most probable pathogen while taking into account the age of the patient and the possibility of underlying disease or anatomic defect.

Sufficient evidence has now accumulated to indicate that combination therapy should not be used in the treatment of bacterial meningitis. In the past combinations of penicillin and chloramphenicol, penicillin and sulfonamides, or penicillin and tetracycline have been used. It is now clear that these generally do more harm than good. Their implementation appears to increase the mortality of the

TABLE 5-1 / Etiologic Agents of Purulent Meningitis in Older Infants, Children, and Adults

Age	Probable Organism
Less than 2 mo.	*E. coli* *Enterobacter* species Other Enterobacteriaceae
2 mo. to 5 yr.	*Haemophilus influenzae* *Neisseria meningitidis* *Diplococcus pneumoniae*
Older than 5 yr.	*D. pneumoniae* *N. meningitidis*

disease and the incidence of neurologic residue without providing a broader spectrum of antimicrobial coverage.

Bacterial meningitis caused by the pneumococcus may be treated with penicillin G in a dosage of 20 to 30 million units daily and continued for 10 to 14 days. Therapy should be instituted rapidly, especially in older persons or when meningitis is associated with alcoholism or is an extension of pneumonia. Case fatality rates in these instances are higher than with any other form of bacterial meningitis.

Meningococcus Meningitis

Since 1968 there has been a nationwide increase in the isolation of group C meningococcus with a decrease in the recovery of group B. The shift in prevalence of serogroups causing disease from primarily group B strains to an overwhelming predominance of group C strains has occurred as a natural phenomenon, as have the periodic outbreaks of disease caused by group A strains in the twentieth century. Studies by Artenstein and his co-workers at the Walter Reed Army Institute of Research [22] have characterized meningococcal infections in military populations over the past eight years. They have clearly shown that most of the disease in the United States is currently due to group C organisms and that virtually all of these organisms are resistant to sulfadiazine. This pattern has emerged despite the fact that sulfadiazine prophylaxis was abandoned in Army training centers in 1964. Although sulfadiazine was an adequate agent for prophylaxis of meningococcal meningitis in the past, the emergence of sulfadiazine resistance in virtually all meningococcal isolates has precluded the use of this drug for prophylactic therapy.

Attempts to replace sulfadiazine with penicillin or erythromycin have been met with only qualified success or failure. Rifampicin has been shown to be effective in the treatment of meningococcal carriers [23], but evidence is now accumulating that the organisms will develop rapid resistance to this drug [24]. At this time it would appear that prophylaxis against meningococcal infection using penicillin or erythromycin is not warranted. Although probably not useful for prophylaxis in large groups, rifampicin may prove valuable in the prophylactic treatment of family contacts. However, at this time the best management of contacts of a patient with meningitis would be careful observation for signs of the disease and the rapid institution of therapy when it appears.

The widespread dissemination of sulfonamide-resistant strains of *N. meningitidis* has lead to an intensive effort to develop potent vaccines to control the spread of the disease in man. The preparation of polysaccharide antigens of high molecular weight from serogroups A, B, and C and a demonstration of the immunogenicity of the A and C products in man have been reported. Further studies have shown that U.S. Army recruits immunized with group C antigen had significantly reduced nasopharyngeal carrier acquisitions of group C organisms as compared with nonimmunized controls. A large field study has demonstrated an 87% reduction in group C disease in vaccinated subjects [25]. The vaccine trial carried out by Artenstein and his co-workers involved over 68,000 military recruits, of which 13,763 received the protective vaccine. This group represented 20% of the entire recruit population, since it was previously shown that immunization of this amount of a given population did not interrupt transmission of group C meningococci among the nonimmunized. Only minor local erythema occurred, and no systemic reactions to the vaccine developed among the 13,763 volunteers. Thirty-eight proved cases of group C meningococcal disease developed in the nonimmunized men, whereas only 1 case occurred in a vaccinated recruit. This 87% reduction in group C disease was statistically significant.

To date at least four large field trials of group C meningococcal vaccine have been carried out involving over 200,000 individuals. The combined results show a reduction in disease consistent with a protective effect of 90% against group-specific organisms. No significant adverse reactions attributable to the vaccine have been observed. The group-specific nature of the protective reaction provided by this group C polysaccharide vaccine is indicated by the observations that all cases of meningococcal disease in the field trials were due to group B organisms and that the attack rate of group B disease was higher among vaccinated recruits than among controls. On occasion the reduction in group C carrier rate among vaccinated recruits was accompanied by an increase in the carrier rate of other serogroups. The wide-scale use of a monovalent vaccine may result in the emergence of other serogroups as causes of disease. A similar phenomenon has been observed with live adenovirus vaccines.

Treatment of meningococcal meningitis is identical to that for pneumococcal meningitis.

Haemophilus Influenzae Meningitis

Ampicillin is now considered to be the drug of choice in meningitis caused by *H. influenzae*. It is generally given to children in a dose of 300 mg. per kilogram of body weight per day in six divided doses; the adult dose is 12 to 16 gm. per day. Ampicillin would be the drug of choice in persons between the ages of two months to 5 years. In the past the combination of penicillin and chloramphenicol was recommended for patients in this age group; such therapy is now outmoded. In a controlled study [26], single-drug ampicillin therapy was shown to be more effective than a combination of ampicillin and chloramphenicol in the three common forms of bacterial meningitis. Analysis of the data from that investigation showed that antibiotic antagonism probably existed in the treatment group that received combination therapy of chloramphenicol plus ampicillin [27]. This has also been shown to be true in experimental pneumococcal meningitis [28].

There have been several recent isolated case reports of failure or relapse of *H. influenzae* meningitis despite ampicillin therapy. Most of these could be shown to be due to inadequate therapy. As the disease process resolves, the dose of ampicillin should be maintained at 300 mg. per kilogram of body weight per day in children, since as the blood–brain barrier reconstitutes itself, the concentration of the antibiotic in the cerebrospinal fluid tends to decline. Duration of treatment is seven to ten days.

Haemophilus influenzae is a rare cause of meningitis in persons over the age of 6 years, and when it occurs one should search for a parameningeal focus of infection. These focuses are usually associated with head injury or immunoglobulin deficiency. This is especially true when the organism is isolated from an adult. The classic studies of Fothergill and Wright [29], in which they described a relationship between age, the occurrence of meningitis due to *H. influenzae,* and the presence of bactericidal antibody against this organism, provided the basis for our current ideas on pathogenesis. In their study of 130 persons they demonstrated that infants had bactericidal activity against this organism in their serum for about two to three months after birth due to maternal antibody. From the age of two to three months until about 3 years this activity was absent; from ages 3 to 10 years there was an increase in the proportion of children who reacquired antibodies against *H. influenzae,* finally reaching about 100% in those 10 years of age and older. These observations correlated very well with the age distribution of *H. influenzae* meningitis, which is highest in infants and children in the age group of two months to 4 years.

A recent report describing a case of *H. influenzae* meningitis in an adult [30] showed that the patient had no bactericidal activity for *H. influenzae* in her serum. Bactericidal activity appeared following the meningitis. These authors then examined the sera from 29 normal adults and found that bactericidal activity was absent in 8 of these individuals (28%). In other cases of adult meningitis due to this organism, antibody activity in the serum was not evaluated. However, a report by Collier, Connor, and Nyhan of *H. influenzae* meningitis in infants less than four months of age (who should be protected by passively transferred antibody) showed that the sera from 4 of the mothers available for examination were deficient in bactericidal activity [31]. This may indicate that the data from 1933 [29] are no longer valid, and in the future *H. influenzae* meningitis may be found with increasing frequency in adults. The trend has already been documented in children [32].

Staphylococcus Meningitis

This is a rare form of meningitis, and there is no consensus regarding its initial therapy. It is frequently fatal, regardless of the treatment employed, and is usually secondary to a bacteremia from an abscess, endocarditis, or a parameningeal focus with direct extension, or it occurs subsequent to a neurosurgical procedure or other trauma to the skull. Initially it will not be known whether the infecting organism is sensitive or resistant to penicillin, so therapy is instituted using an agent that is effective against both types of staphylococci: one of the semisynthetic penicillins, oxacillin, 12 gm. per day, or nafcillin, 20 gm. per day, should be administered intravenously as a constant infusion or in divided doses every 4 to 6 hours. If the staphylococcus is subsequently shown to be sensitive to penicillin, therapy may be changed to penicillin G, 20 to 30 million units per day, given intravenously. Therapy should be continued for at least ten days to two weeks.

Gram-Negative Organisms Causing Meningitis

In most cases the diagnosis is based on the finding of an extrameningeal focus of infection and gram-negative bacilli in the cerebrospinal fluid. The species of organism may only be inferred unless the extrameningeal infection is one which has been established for some time and the organism identified; therefore, it is necessary to provide wide-spectrum coverage on an empirical basis. The least toxic combination of drugs which provides the widest antimicrobial spectrum is ampicillin and gentamicin. The latter drug is chosen in preference to the other aminoglycosides since it is less ototoxic and nephrotoxic and encompasses the therapeutic spectrum of the polymyxins. Ampicillin should be administered as described for *H. influenzae* meningitis. Gentamicin should be given in the amount of 5 to 6 mg. per kilogram of body weight per 24 hours intramuscularly, divided into four doses, and 0.5 to 1 mg. per day should be administered intrathecally. Treatment may be altered if the response is poor or as indicated by subsequent sensitivity testing. If the infecting species is a *Pseudomonas* not sensitive to gentamicin, then polymyxin B or colistin may be given intramuscularly together with intrathecal administration of polymyxin

B. Polymyxin B sulfate may be given in a dose of 0.5 to 2.5 mg. per kilogram of body weight per day in patients with normal renal function. For intravenous administration the calculated dose is dissolved in 200 to 500 ml. of 5% dextrose in water and infused over a sixty-minute period, or two infusions 12 hours apart may be given instead. For intramuscular administration the daily dosage should be administered every 6 hours. Colistin (polymyxin E) is usually administered in a dosage of 3 to 5 mg. per kilogram of body weight given in two to four divided doses. Polymyxin B may be given intrathecally by dissolving 2 to 3 mg. of the drug in 10 ml. of isotonic saline and injecting it over a ten-minute period after the removal of 10 ml. of cerebrospinal fluid.

Therapy in Persons Allergic to Penicillin

The treatment of meningitis in persons allergic to penicillin will depend to a certain extent on the manifestations of allergy to the drug. It is always dangerous to administer an allergen to a person known to be sensitive to the agent; however, in the case of fulminant meningitis due to the pneumococcus or meningococcus the risks of not using penicillin may outweigh the risks of the allergic manifestations of the drug. If an allergic reaction develops during treatment and the reaction is mild, such as itching or rash, then penicillin may be continued and the allergic symptoms treated with antihistamines or hydrocortisone equivalents. However, when the allergic manifestations are not known and there is a reasonable expectation that anaphylaxis might occur, a good alternative would be chloramphenicol. Chloramphenicol penetrates the meninges better than any other antibiotic, and it is administered at a dose of 75 to 100 mg. per kilogram of body weight per day to a maximum of 4 gm. per day. The idiosyncratic aplastic reaction to chloramphenicol occurs about once in 25,000 persons and is not a contraindication to the use of the antibiotic in this situation. This reaction is anticipated by a rise in the serum iron concentration about one week before the aplastic crisis is manifested peripherally. Erythromycin may be used as an alternate drug, although it penetrates the blood–brain barrier only in concentrations of about 8 to 20% of those in the serum and is inferior to chloramphenicol in this respect.

REFERENCES

1. Fosson, A. R., and Fine, R. H. Neonatal meningitis: Presentation and discussion of 21 cases. *Clin. Pediat.* (Phila.) 7:404, 1968.
2. Overall, J. C. Neonatal bacterial meningitis: Analysis of predisposing

factors and outcome compared with matched control subjects. *J. Pediat.* 76:499, 1970.

3. Mace, J. W., Peters, E. R., and Mathies, A. W., Jr. Cranial bruits in purulent meningitis in childhood. *New Eng. J. Med.* 278:1429, 1968.
4. Dowling, H. F. *The Acute Bacterial Diseases, Their Diagnosis and Treatment.* Philadelphia: Saunders, 1948. Pp. 202–226.
5. Feldman, H. A. Recent developments in the therapy and control of meningococcal infections. *D. M.*, February, 1966.
6. Vedros, N. A., Hunter, D. H., and Rust, J. H., Jr. Studies on immunity in meningococcal meningitis. *Milit. Med.* 131:1413, 1966.
7. Artenstein, M. S., Rust, J. H., Hunter, D. H., Lamson, T. H., and Buescher, E. L. Acute respiratory disease and meningococcal infection in army recruits. *J.A.M.A.* 201:1004, 1967.
8. Austrian, R. The role of toxemia and of neural injury in the outcome of pneumococcal meningitis. *Amer. J. Med. Sci.* 247:257, 1964.
9. Lepper, M. H., Sweet, L. K., and Dowling, H. F. The treatment of meningococci infections with sulfadiazine and sulfamerazine. *J.A.M.A.* 123:134, 1943.
10. Welch, K., and Pollay, M. Perfusion of particles through arachnoid villi of the monkey. *Amer. J. Physiol.* 201:651, 1961.
11. Penner, A., and Bernheim, A. I. Studies in the pathogenesis of experimental dysentery intoxication: Production of lesions by introduction of toxin into the cerebral ventricles. *J. Exp. Med.* 111:145, 1960.
12. Atwood, R. P., and Kass, E. H. Relationship of body temperature to the lethal action of bacterial endotoxin. *J. Clin. Invest.* 43:151, 1964.
13. Palmerio, C., Zetterstrom, B., Shammash, J., Euchbaum, E., Frank, E., and Fine, J. Denervation of the abdominal viscera for the treatment of traumatic shock. *New Eng. J. Med.* 269:709, 1963.
14. Lillehei, R. C., Lonerbeam, J. K., and Bloch, J. H. Physiology and therapy of bacteremic shock: Experimental and clinical observations. *Amer. J. Cardiol.* 12:599, 1963.
15. Kass, E. H., Atwood, R. P., and Porter, P. J. Observations of Lethal Action of Bacterial Endotoxin. In W. Braun and M. Landy (Eds.), *Bacterial Endotoxin.* New Brunswick, N. J.: Rutgers University Press, 1964.
16. Hardman, J. M., and Earle, K. M. Meningococcal infections: A review of 200 fatal cases. *J. Neuropath. Exp. Neurol.* 26:119, 1967.
17. Ferguson, J. H., and Chapman, O. D. Fulminating meningococcal infections and the so-called Waterhouse-Friederichsen syndrome. *Amer. J. Path.* 24:763, 1948.
18. Ducker, T. B., and Simmons, R. L. The pathogenesis of meningitis. *Arch. Neurol.* (Chicago) 18:123, 1968.
19. Simmons, R. L., Ducker, T. B., Martin, A. M., Anderson, R. W., and Noyes, H. E. The role of the central nervous system in septic shock: I. Pathologic changes following intraventricular and intracisternal endotoxin in the dog. *Ann. Surg.* 167:145, 1968.
20. Gilbert, R. P. Mechanisms of the hemodynamic effects of endotoxin. *Physiol. Rev.* 40:245, 1960.
21. Penner, A., and Bernheim, A. I. Studies in the pathogenesis of experimental dysentery intoxication. *J. Exp. Med.* 76:271, 1942.

22. Artenstein, M. S., Schneider, H., and Tingley, M. D. Meningococcal infections. *Bull. W.H.O.* 45:275, 1971.
23. Deal, W. B., and Sanders, E. Efficacy of Rifampin in treatment of meningococcal carriers. *New Eng. J. Med.* 281:641, 1969.
24. Beam, W. E., Newberg, N. R., Devine, L. F., Pierce, W. E., and Davies, J. A. The effects of Rifampin on the nasopharyngeal carriage of *Neisseria meningitidis* in a military population. *J. Infect. Dis.* 124:39, 1971.
25. Artenstein, M. S., Gold, R., Zimmerly, J. G., Wylie, F. A., Schneider, H., and Harkins, C. Prevention of meningococcal disease by group C polysaccharide vaccine. *New Eng. J. Med.* 282:417, 1970.
26. Wehrle, P. F., Mathies, A. W., and Leedom, J. M. The critically ill child: Management of acute bacterial meningitis. *Pediatrics* 44:991, 1969.
27. Mathies, A. W., Leedom, J. M., Ivier, D., Wehrle, P. F., and Portnoy, B. Antibiotic antagonism in bacterial meningitis. *Antimicrob. Agents Chemother.* 218, 1968.
28. Wallace, J. F., Smith, R. H., and Petersdorf, R. G. Studies on the pathogenesis of meningitis: VI. Antagonism between penicillin and chloramphenicol in experimental meningitis. *J. Lab. Clin. Med.* 70:408, 1967.
29. Fothergill, L. D., and Wright, J. Influenzal meningitis: The relation of age incidence to the bactericidal power of blood against the causal organism. *J. Immun.* 24:273, 1933.
30. Norden, C. W., Callerame, M. L., and Baum, J. *Hemophilus influenzae* meningitis in an adult. *New Eng. J. Med.* 282:190, 1970.
31. Collier, A. M., Connor, J. D., and Nyhan, W. L. Systemic infection with *Hemophilus influenzae* in very young infants. *J. Pediat.* 70:539, 1967.
32. Michaels, R. H. Increase in influenzal meningitis. *New Eng. J. Med.* 285:666, 1971.

6 / URINARY TRACT INFECTIONS

J. Joseph Marr

INFECTIONS of the urinary tract are among the most frequent problems treated by the physician, yet their propensity to recur, despite seemingly adequate therapy, makes them a most vexing problem in an office practice. These recurrences are generally due to reinfection by a different organism except when an anatomic or functional abnormality of the urinary tract is present. In these instances recurrence is usually due to the persistence of the original organism which has maintained itself in the renal parenchyma to emerge within a few weeks after chemotherapy has been discontinued. Therefore, it is of some importance to know if renal involvement exists or whether the infection is confined to the lower urinary tract. Numerous studies carried out in the past ten years have shown that the risk of pyelonephritis varies markedly with the particular group of persons studied. As a result, it has become possible to predict with some confidence the probable pathology and natural history of the disease in an individual.

The majority of urinary infections occur in women, the incidence increasing in a linear fashion with age, beginning in adolescence until the sixth decade of life, when there is a more rapid increment. In men the situation is quite different. The incidence is relatively low until the sixth decade, when prostatic hypertrophy and the attendant obstruction bring about a steep increase in the number of cases. Infections in men under the age of 50 are uncommon and imply anatomic or functional anomaly of the genitourinary system.

There are two groups of individuals which deserve particular attention by the practitioner of medicine; these are children and pregnant women. The common denominator between them is asymptomatic infection.

Large-scale studies in various areas of the world have documented the prevalence of asymptomatic bacteriuria. It may indeed be one of the most common infections of the European and American populations. The investigations of Kunin and co-workers [1, 2] have shown that the prevalence of bacteriuria is 5% during the elementary and secondary school years. The significance of this finding is underscored by the fact that about 14% of those with infection showed calicectasis and 19% had vesicoureteral reflux. Other studies by Smellie et al. [3] have demonstrated renal scarring in infected children with a resumption of kidney growth following adequate therapy. The evidence at this time indicates that young girls with bacteriuria, whether symptomatic or not, should be adequately treated and followed with repeated urine cultures for a year in order to be certain of a cure.

Recent reports by Kunin [4, 5], published at the conclusion of his long-term study on bacteriuria in schoolgirls, have documented the epidemiology and natural history of this problem. The participants had bacteriuria uncomplicated by major urologic abnormalities, and most recurrences were either asymptomatic or associated with lower urinary tract complaints. The cumulative prevalence of bacteriuria, as mentioned above, was about 5% for girls in the elementary and secondary school years. The yearly overall conversion rate was 0.43%. This information, together with the known frequency of recurrence of bacteriuria, substantiates the view that many of the urinary tract infections seen in adult women may have had their inception during childhood.

The data regarding the recurrence of infection in treated individuals are perhaps the most interesting of the entire long-term study. The problem of recurrence is a difficult one to evaluate, since bacteriuria in schoolgirls is a common phenomenon, is often asymptomatic, and frequently undergoes long periods of remission following a specific course of therapy. In this respect it appears to be a benign form of urinary colonization. However, in any population of bacteriuric girls there will also be many who have frequent symptomatic recurrences of infection, which may sometimes be manifested as pyelonephritis. Some of these individuals demonstrate loss of renal function despite the fact that their infections are asymptomatic and there are no obstructive lesions evident.

Recurrent infections are most common during the first two years following antimicrobial therapy, with the risk of recurrence decreasing thereafter. Moreover, there appears to be a difference in recurrence rate between Negro girls and Caucasian girls. With regard to the latter, each treatment brings about cure (long-term remission) in about 20 to 25%. This is irrespective of the number of preceding treatments, even in girls with as many as ten or more preceding courses of therapy. Therefore, the number of girls requiring multiple treatments decreases in a logarithmic fashion with time. Although the number of Negro girls in this study was small, it appears that the recurrence rate is less with this group. With each course of therapy about 40% of the population under treatment is brought into long-term remission. The same results are obtained when white and Negro girls are matched for both age and socioeconomic status. The results of these studies also show that recurrences, or the number of treatments required during a given period of years, are much greater for young girls than for older girls. It is of interest that differences in socioeconomic class among girls of a given race did not have an effect on the rate of recurrence. More important, the rate of recurrence was also not different between girls found to have vesicoureteral reflux and girls without this finding. Race and age appear to be the most significant determinants of the rate of recurrence of bacteriuria.

If one examines the rapidity with which urinary tract infections recur following treatment, two patterns are seen to emerge. In those individuals who have a relapse of the original infection, evidence of recurrence usually appears within the first three to six months after the last episode. Relapse can be differentiated conclusively from reinfection by demonstrating that the infecting organism is of the same serotype as that previously recovered. These individuals usually relapse because of insufficient treatment of the initiating infection or the presence of an anatomic abnormality or a calculus. In the second group, which under most conditions is by far the larger, about 80% of recurrence is a result of reinfection by an organism different from the one previously present. These organisms usually come from the gastrointestinal tract. This is of some importance when one considers the distribution of a drug within the body when treating a urinary tract infection. For example, sulfonamides are found in the gastrointestinal tract and excreted in the stool; thus reinfecting organisms will already be resistant to these drugs. On the other hand, nitrofurantoin is excreted to a very small extent in the stool, so that reinfecting organisms remain sensitive to this drug and it retains its value in the treatment of chronic recurrent urinary tract infections for those patients who can tolerate the drug.

When one examines the rate at which late recurrences, i.e., reinfection, occur, it becomes evident that the longer a girl is free of infection, the less chance there is for her to have a recurrence. For example, the risk of acquiring bacteriuria within one year after treatment is about 50%, whereas if one remains free of bacteriuria during that first year the risks of acquiring it during the second year drop to 27%. If one remains free of bacteriuria during the first two years, the risk of acquiring it during the third year falls to 18%. During the fourth year and years thereafter, the risk is about 5 to 8%. These rates are, nevertheless, much higher than the rate of emergence of bacteriuria noted in the general population of schoolgirls mentioned earlier; that rate is 0.43% per year. Previous bacteriuric episodes therefore appear to distinguish cases from the general population of schoolgirls and define a group of girls exposed at high risk to infection later in life. These individuals are at a significantly greater risk of reacquiring bacteriuria after marriage and pregnancy.

Acquisition of bacteriuria and symptomatic infection within three months of marriage will be found both in women who were free of infection for several years as well as in those who were infected within one year before marriage. Bacteriuria is also common in association with pregnancy, even in women who have been free of infection for a long period of time. The association between sexual activity and bacteriuria is also emphasized by a study of women in whom recurrences developed after they had been free of infection for more than three years. The immediate precipitating event could be clearly defined in 65% of these as being related to recent marriage, pregnancy, or sexual intercourse.

The corollary to the above is that bacteriuria in young boys is of even more importance than it is in girls. The investigations cited above, as well as others [6], have confirmed that bacteriuria in boys is rare (0.03%) but that when it does occur, it almost invariably is associated with an anatomic abnormality and some degree of obstruction. Management of young boys with a urinary tract infection requires adequate chemotherapy and subsequent urologic investigation to determine if a correctable abnormality exists.

The therapeutic implications of the foregoing are evident. There is no doubt that bacteriuria is associated with the tendency to symptomatic renal disease. This is clear from the studies mentioned and also from the study of bacteriuric women who become pregnant [7]. In pregnancy the data are quite clear that bacteriuric women have a higher risk of later developing symptomatic pyelonephritis than do nonbacteriuric women; elimination of bacteriuria gives virtually complete freedom from clinical pyelonephritis.

During pregnancy as many as 5 to 7% of women will have asymptomatic infections; an additional 1 to 2% will develop bacteriuria during gestation, usually in the last trimester [8]. A significant number of these women will develop symptomatic pyelonephritis, either during the pregnancy or within a few months postpartum. Several controlled studies of treated and placebo-treated subjects have demonstrated a 20 to 45% incidence of pyelonephritis in the placebo group [9, 10] as compared to less than 5% in the treated group. There is also an increased incidence of abortions and prematurity among pregnant women with asymptomatic infection and a higher incidence of hypertension and chronic renal disease later in life [11]. The effectiveness of therapeutic intervention in these patients was well demonstrated by the study of Brumfitt [12], in which he showed that no fewer than 25% of pregnant bacteriuric women develop pyelonephritis, but when the organism was eliminated by treatment the frequency fell to about 3%. It is reasonable to conclude that screening for bacteriuria should be done early in pregnancy and continued throughout the period of gestation. When found, it should be treated vigorously with the least toxic drugs available whether symptoms are present or not. Finally, patients found to have infections should be followed with several urine cultures after delivery and treated if bacteriuria returns. This last point should not be overlooked, since 50 to 80% of untreated women will have persisting bacteriuria during the year following delivery [13, 14]. Of those who are treated and whose urine is cleared of organisms during the pregnancy, about 20% will have a recurrence during the next two to four years [15].

In summary, although there is insufficient evidence to establish a causal relationship between asymptomatic bacteriuria and chronic renal disease, hyposthenuria, radiologic evidence of pyelonephritis, and bacteremia, such an association is likely. There is, nevertheless, adequate documentation of the causative role of asymptomatic bacteriuria to reversible radiographic renal lesions, pyelonephritis of pregnancy, and postcatheterization bacteremia. Therefore, patients who have recently suffered a renal infection and pregnant women constitute a particularly vulnerable group in whom bacteriuria demands eradication. The same is true for those who are to undergo instrumentation or manipulation of the genitourinary tract [16].

DEMONSTRATION OF SIGNIFICANT BACTERIURIA

The demonstration of bacteria in a single unspun clean-voided urine specimen may not be sufficient evidence on which to initiate therapy, since many persons with this finding will have sterile urine on subsequent cultures. However, if 100,000 organisms per milliliter are cultured on two or three successive attempts, then the person must be considered as being infected whether symptoms are present or not. Examination should be carried out immediately after obtaining the specimen, since contaminants may overgrow the causative organism or give a false impression of an infected urine when there were but few organisms present at the time of voiding. Casts will also break apart if the urine is allowed to stand. Culture of the urine is the most important diagnostic procedure and should be performed as rapidly as possible. For proper therapy the causative organism should be identified and antibiotic susceptibility studies done.

Because of the great variability in sensitivity to antimicrobial agents, general rules may not be applicable. Optimal results will be obtained by employing the drug dictated by antibiotic sensitivity testing of the patient's own organism. Some guidelines for therapy are presented below.

THERAPY OF URINARY TRACT INFECTIONS

Infections of the urinary tract may be conceptually divided into those involving the upper tract (kidney) and the lower tract. Either form may be additionally described as simple or complicated, the latter term generally implying a chronic recurrent infection. Simple infections, most of which are asymptomatic, respond quickly and easily to therapy. Chronic or recurrent infections are eradicated only with difficulty and are frequently associated with an anatomic abnormality, e.g., calculus, stricture, or reflux. Most chronic infections will be associated with obstruction of the lower or upper urinary tract, instrumentation, indwelling catheters, or neurogenic bladder dysfunction with a significant residual. The most common pathogen is *Escherichia coli,* accounting for 80 to 90% of all infections. Chronic infections may be due to *E. coli* that are frequently resistant to most antibiotics, but they also may be caused by a variety of other gram-negative organisms—notably *Klebsiella-Enterobacter* species, *Proteus,* or *Pseudomonas.* Gram-positive organisms account for less than 10% of all infections.

Asymptomatic Bacteriuria and Simple Infections

These are usually caused by *E. coli* or *P. mirabilis* sensitive to most antimicrobial agents. The sulfonamides, because of their low cost, efficacy, and absence of significant side effects, are quite adequate. They have the additional benefit of being nontoxic to the fetus and therefore very acceptable for treatment of asymptomatic bacteriuria of pregnancy. Despite their wide antibacterial spectrum, they seldom produce an imbalance of intestinal flora and diarrhea. The antibacterial differences among the sulfonamides are slight, so that the choice depends to a considerable degree upon the rate at which the drug is acetylated and excreted. Sulfisoxazole is the single agent most often used and is probably among the most effective. In 24 hours about 95% of the drug will be excreted in the urine, and only a third of this will be acetylated. Thus the major portion remains in the active form, making this among the most soluble of the sulfa drugs. The inactive acetylated derivative tends to crystallize in an acid urine and may produce obstruction; for this reason the urine should be alkalinized when sulfonamides are given. Triple sulfa mixtures take advantage of the fact that each drug behaves as though it were in solution alone with respect to its solubility, yet the antibacterial effects are additive. This combination was designed to circumvent the problem of crystalluria but is probably not superior to sulfisoxazole alone. The usual course of therapy is ten days and may be repeated if the infection recurs. A repeat culture and sensitivity testing should be done at the third or fourth day of treatment to be certain that the drug is effective. The use of the long-acting sulfonamides, such as Kynex, Midicel, and Madribon, has been associated with serious toxic and hypersensitivity reactions and cannot be recommended.

A valuable alternate agent that is relatively nontoxic is nitrofurantoin. Blood concentrations are very low, but bactericidal concentrations are attained in the urine and the renal lymph as well. In contrast to the sulfonamides, acidification of the urine aids antibacterial activity. Most organisms are sensitive to the drug, with the exception of *Pseudomonas* species. The usual dosage is 100 to 150 mg. four times a day. Nitrofurantoin may produce a brown color in the urine, and patients should be told to expect it. The drug is best avoided when renal insufficiency is present, since under these conditions it does not enter the urine and a polyneuritis has been described when significant concentrations accumulate in the blood.

When primary treatment with the above drugs fails, then penicillin G, ampicillin, or tetracycline are useful. Penicillin G administered in doses of 800,000 units every 6 hours will effect a urine concentration of 100 μg. per milliliter; it is an extremely safe drug and worthy of a trial, even when sensitivities are equivocal, since concentrations may be achieved in the urine which are far higher than those obtained in disc sensitivity testing. Ampicillin may be given as a 500 mg. dose every 6 hours. Tetracycline should be avoided in the treatment of asymptomatic bacteriuria of pregnancy because of its possible effects on the fetus and the occasional instances of liver necrosis seen in pregnant women. This latter complication is usually a result of intravenous therapy. Usual dosage is 1 to 2 gm. per day in four doses.

Failure of the above regimens in an infection caused by a sensitive organism is generally an indication of an anatomic abnormality of the urinary tract or renal parenchymal infection or both.

Upper Urinary Tract Infection (Acute Pyelonephritis)

In the presence of clinical evidence of acute pyelonephritis, consideration must be given to the concentration of the drug in the renal tissue as well as in the urine. This is a topic of considerable controversy, but some promising data have emerged from cannulation of the renal lymphatics in animals and determinations of the antibiotic concentrations therein. However, at this time the choice of an agent must still be based upon the accumulated clinical experience with acute pyelonephritis. The agent selected should be bactericidal, since organisms residing in the renal medulla are metabolizing slowly and perhaps are protected partially from the immune response by the inactivation of the fourth component of complement due to the high concentration of ammonia. Intramuscular ampicillin, 500 mg. every 6 hours, would appear at this writing to be the agent of choice since high blood and urine concentrations are obtained. The majority of cases of acute pyelonephritis are due to *E. coli,* which are sensitive to ampicillin in adequate dosage. If the organism is resistant to the drug, it may be treated with one of the agents described in the following section.

Chronic Recurrent Urinary Tract Infections

Chronic bacteriuria can arise from diverse sources. Bladder dysfunction and urine retention may allow persistence of bacteria, and infections established in the prostate or in the paraurethral apparatus in the female may result in recurring infection. The typical patient with chronic bacteriuria is a woman who has had episodes of reinfection over a period of years; the source is usually *E. coli* from the feces. These strains are generally sensitive to most antibiotics. A recent study of 89 women who suffered from chronic bacteriuria for a mean duration of twelve years [17] showed that about half of them had renal involvement each time the urine became infected. This conclusion was based on the finding of elevated antibody titers to the infecting organism. Radiologic investigation indicated that significant renal changes had occurred in half of these individuals. Thus the situation in adult women is somewhat analogous to that in schoolgirls, although the etiologic factors of reflux and progressive scarring have not been shown to be operable in adult women. Each episode of infection in the adult is usually due to reinfection (as opposed to recurrence) and suggests an impairment of the defense mechanisms of the lower tract.

Chronic bacteriuria in the older male does not appear to have the same origin and is less likely to cause renal damage. The most frequent predisposing factor is obstructive uropathy, usually due to prostatic hypertrophy. A study by Freeman et al. [18] showed that whereas infections in women and children were almost always due to *E. coli* and *P. mirabilis,* only 34% of males with chronic bacteriuria had *E. coli* as the causative organism. This suggests that the organism was acquired in the hospital, perhaps following instrumentation or surgery.

The decision as to which patients with chronic urinary tract infections should be treated is still a matter of some dispute, since there is no agreement as to how often chronic bacteriuria confined to the lower tract ascends to involve the kidney. However, experience with bacteriuria of long duration in adult women has shown that chronic active pyelonephritis and renal damage are frequent concomitants. Treatment of this group is, in the author's opinion, indicated. As mentioned above, this sequence has also been shown to occur in children and pregnant women. Bacteriuria in elderly males is often benign, and at this time there is little evidence to support the view that long-term prophylaxis prevents renal deterioration in these patients. Caution would dictate, however, that elderly males (or anyone) with a debilitating disease should be treated lest gram-negative bacteremia supervene.

The following is a consensus view of modes of therapy for chronic bacteriuria. Recurrent infections should be treated with an antibiotic demonstrated to be efficacious by culture and sensitivity testing. The agent should be bactericidal, and the length of therapy should be ten to fourteen days. Current evidence [19, 20] indicates that prolongation of therapy for up to six weeks does not improve the result. Ampicillin, as described previously, will often be adequate; however, in recurrent bacteriuria (especially in males) resistant organisms will occasionally exist and require more intensive therapy. Alternate drugs which may be used are:

colistin, 2.5 to 5 mg./kg.	in divided doses
gentamicin, 1 to 2 mg./kg.	in divided doses
kanamycin, 10 to 15 mg./kg.	in divided doses
polymyxin B, 1 to 1.5 mg./kg.	in divided doses

After treatment of the recurrences, patients who have had more than three to four reinfections should be placed on long-term suppressive therapy. Both nitrofurantoin and methenamine mandelate (Mandelamine) have been used, with about equal effectiveness. The rationale for long-term suppressive therapy lies in the studies of Kunin [4, 5] on recurrence of infection and the observation that the kidney has the capacity to rid itself of gram-negative bacteria over a few weeks as long as it is not continually reinfected via ascending spread from the bladder. The value of methenamine mandelate is due to the facts that organisms do not become resistant to it (as in the case of the antibiotics just mentioned) and it renders the urine an unsuitable medium for growth. Methenamine mandelate is the methoxamine salt of mandelic acid; both of these compounds are bactericidal. The former liberates formaldehyde in an acid urine, and the latter is intrinsically effective. The usual dose is 1 gm. four times a day. Since the urine must be acid for the drug to be effective, ascorbic acid (1 gm. four times a day) is generally given along with it.

Newer Antimicrobial Agents

The antibacterial spectrum of carbenicillin is similar to that for ampicillin; however, it has the decided advantage of being effective against *P. aeruginosa* and *Proteus* species resistant to ampicillin. It is not efficacious against Klebsiellae and is less active against gram-positive cocci than other penicillins. The drug is not absorbed to any appreciable degree when given orally; intramuscular injections give peak serum concentrations in 1 hour. The major use of carbenicillin is in the treatment of urinary tract infections, and its place in systemic infections with *Pseudomonas* species will not be discussed. The pharmacologic attributes are those of the other semisynthetic penicillins, and it may be used in the presence of renal failure since this is a relative contraindication to the use of the polymyxins and aminoglycoside antibiotics. Depending upon the preparation of carbenicillin, it may contain from 4 to 7 mEq. of sodium per gram, which may be of significance in persons with renal impairment or cardiac failure. The usual dose for urinary tract infections is 1 gm. every 6 hours. Since resistance to this agent develops rapidly, especially when the dosage is inadequate, it should be reserved for the treatment of infections due to *Pseudomonas* or *Proteus* species resistant to other antibiotics or when deteriorating renal function has become a significant factor in the management of the patient.

Gentamicin is a relatively new aminoglycoside which is active against nearly all of the gram-negative organisms of clinical interest, and at this time it is effective against more hospital pathogens than any other single antibiotic. In order to minimize the appearance of resistant strains, it should not be used unless absolutely indicated. Its primary clinical value is in the treatment of infections due to *Proteus* and *Pseudomonas* species. Very high levels may be obtained in the urine at doses of 0.5 to 1.0 mg. per kilogram of body weight divided into a three-times-daily regimen. As with the other aminoglycoside antibiotics (streptomycin, kanamycin), alkalinization of the urine is important since the effectiveness of the drug increases markedly as the pH increases. Since there is no major extrarenal route for excretion, it must be administered cautiously in the presence of renal failure. Clinical isolates resistant to the other aminoglycoside antibiotics frequently will not display resistance to gentamicin.

Cephalexin represents an attempt to combine the side chain of ampicillin with the nucleus of a cephalosporin in order to gain the advantages of both drugs. It appears to hold great promise on the basis of experimental studies and accumulating clinical experience. It is a cephalosporin which can be administered orally, and its primary use is in the treatment of urinary tract infections. About half of an ingested dose appears in the urine within 2 hours.

VESICOURETERAL REFLUX

The controversy that vesicoureteral reflux has generated over many years makes it worthy of separate mention. Reflux is commonly found in children with urinary tract infections. The results of a number of studies indicate that the rate is about 20 to 30% in symptomatic children, and renal scarring and diminished size of the kidneys can be found in association with it. Reflux appears to diminish in frequency with age, even in patients who present with symptomatic infection. A study by Baker et al. [21] showed that 26% of the children examined had reflux, but only 5% of adult patients seen on a urologic service had this problem. The studies of Kunin, already described, also showed a similar tendency for reflux to become less common with age. All of this indicates that reflux often disappears spontaneously, and more reports of this spontaneous disappearance might be expected as conservative management increases. There is now a growing tendency among urologic surgeons not to operate unless reflux persists for more than a year or is associated with evidence of hydronephrosis or renal damage [22].

PREVENTION OF HOSPITAL-ACQUIRED URINARY TRACT INFECTIONS

These are the most frequent hospital-acquired infections and are nearly always associated with instrumentation or catheterization. At times catheters are indispensable for therapy, but the indications should be quite clear. They should be placed using aseptic technique and removed as soon as possible. Repeated properly done catheterizations are preferable to an indwelling catheter. When an indwelling catheter is required, the incidence of significant infection will be lessened if a triple-lumen catheter is employed and the bladder continuously irrigated with a solution of 40 mg. neomycin and 20 mg. polymyxin B per liter of normal saline. An alternate, though less effective, method is the use of a closed urinary drainage system with a disposable sterile bag and spigot attachment to permit semipermanent use. The catheter should not be irrigated unless obstruction is suspected. Bags are drained with care taken not to contaminate the spigot. After a catheter is removed, a urine culture must be obtained and treatment instituted for significant persisting bacteriuria.

REFERENCES

1. Kunin, C. M., Deutscher, R., and Paquin, A. Urinary tract infection in school children: An epidemiologic, clinical and laboratory study. *Medicine* 43:91, 1964.
2. Kunin, C. M. Emergence of bacteriuria, proteinuria, and symptomatic urinary tract infections among a population of school girls followed for seven years. *Pediatrics* 41:968, 1968.
3. Smellie, J. M., Hodson, C. J., Edwards, D., and Normand, I. C. S. Clinical and radiological features of urinary infection in childhood. *Brit. Med. J.* 2:1222, 1964.
4. Kunin, C. M. The natural history of recurrence of bacteriuria in school girls. *New Eng. J. Med.* 282:1443, 1970.
5. Kunin, C. M. A 10 year study of bacteriuria in school girls: Final report of bacteriologic, urologic, and epidemiologic findings. *J. Infect. Dis.* 122:382, 1970.
6. Kunin, C. M., and Paquin, A. J. Frequency and Natural History of Urinary Tract Infection in School Children. In E. H. Kass (Ed.), *Progress in Pyelonephritis*. Philadelphia: Davis, 1965. Pp. 33–44.
7. Norden, C. W., and Kass, E. H. Bacteriuria of pregnancy: A critical reappraisal. *Ann. Rev. Med.* 19:431, 1968.
8. Whalley, P. Bacteriuria of pregnancy. *Amer. J. Obstet. Gynec.* 97:723, 1967.
9. Pathak, U. N., Tang, K., Williams, L. L., and Stuart, K. L. Bacteriuria of pregnancy: Results of treatment. *J. Infect. Dis.* 120:91, 1969.
10. Kincaid-Smith, P. Bacteriuria in Pregnancy. In E. H. Kass (Ed.), *Progress in Pyelonephritis*. Philadelphia: Davis, 1965. Pp. 11–26.
11. Stuart, K. L., Cummins, G. T. M., and Chin, W. A. Bacteriuria, prematurity and the hypertensive disorders of pregnancy. *Brit. Med. J.* 1:554, 1965.
12. Brumfitt, W. In O. M. Wrong (Ed.), *Fourth Symposium for Advanced Medicine*. London, 1968. P. 51.

13. Whalley, P. J., Martin, F. G., and Peters, P. C. Significance of asymptomatic bacteriuria detected during pregnancy. *J.A.M.A.* 193:879, 1965.
14. Cobbs, C. G., Strickler, J. C., McGovern, J. M., and Kaye, D. The postpartum renal status of women with untreated asymptomatic bacteriuria during pregnancy. *Amer. J. Obstet. Gynec.* 99:221, 1967.
15. Leigh, D. A., Gruneberg, R. D., and Brumfitt, W. Long-term follow-up of bacteriuria in pregnancy. *Lancet* 1:603, 1968.
16. Kass, E. H., and Zinner, S. H. Bacteriuria and renal disease. *J. Infect. Dis.* 120:27, 1969.
17. Brumfitt, W., Pursell, R., Ormonde, N. W. H., Murdoch, J. M., and Wallace, E. Chronic bacteriuria due to *Escherichia coli:* II. Correlation of microbiological, radiological, and biochemical findings with the clinical results. *J. Infect. Dis.* 120:87, 1969.
18. Freeman, R. B., Bromer, L., Brancato, F., Cohen, S., Garfield, C. F., Griep, R. J., Hinman, E. J., Richardson, J. A., Thurm, R. H., Urner, C., and Smith, W. Prevention of recurrent bacteriuria with continuous chemotherapy. *Ann. Intern. Med.* 69:655, 1968.
19. Kincaid-Smith, P., and Fairley, K. F. Controlled trial comparing effect of two and six weeks' treatment in recurrent urinary tract infection. *Brit. Med. J.* 2:145, 1969.
20. Brumfitt, W., and Reeves, D. S. Recent developments in the treatment of urinary tract infection. *J. Infect. Dis.* 120:61, 1969.
21. Baker, R., Maxted, W., Maylath, J., and Shuman, I. Relation of age, sex, and infection to reflux: Data indicating high spontaneous cure rate in pediatric patients. *J. Urol.* 95:27, 1966.
22. O'Donnell, B., Moloney, M. A., and Lynch, V. Vesico-ureteric reflux in infants and children: Results of "supervision," chemotherapy and surgery. *Brit. Med. J.* 16:6, 1969.

7 / GRAM-NEGATIVE SEPTICEMIA

Malcolm T. Foster, Jr., and
Owen S. Kantor

FROM ITS DESCRIPTION as a syndrome in 1951, gram-negative septicemia has escalated in importance. A large volume of literature has provided a good clinical description of the syndrome and its epidemiology. Unfortunately the pathophysiology is not completely understood and is often contradictory due to the lack of an animal model which parallels the human disease.

Gram-negative septicemia may occur in the very young or in the elderly, in postpartum women or in men after a transurethral resection. In patients compromised by disease or by therapy, any one of a host of bacteria may cause the syndrome. Even within a well-defined subgroup—for instance, *Escherichia coli* septicemia complicating transurethral resections—the clinical manifestations, the underlying pathophysiology, and indeed the outcome may be dissimilar. Gram-negative septicemia is a clinical syndrome, therefore, with multiple expressions and physiological mechanisms that are poorly understood.

Bacterial invasion of the bloodstream may be self-limited and transient, or it may be intermittent or continuous. Septicemia implies a bacteremia which is symptomatic. The most common symptoms are fever and chills. Mild hypotension is often observed early; it, too, can be self-limiting and can be transient, intermittent, or continuous. Gram-negative bacteria account for most instances of bacteremia or septicemia recognized in hospitals today. The patient with gram-negative septicemia and shock will develop the abrupt onset of fever; chills; hypotension; tachycardia; weak, thready pulses; cool, clammy skin; peripheral cyanosis; oliguria; tachypnea; and alterations of the sensorium. A few patients will appear warm and pink, maintain a good urinary output, and experience mild or no changes in mentation. Some patients will pass from this stage of warm shock into the more classic picture.

For many patients the clinical picture of gram-negative septicemia with shock is highly variable. Most will have fever, although an occasional patient will be hypothermic. Chills may be absent in as many as half of the patients, particularly in the elderly and in patients with leukemia. Some patients will develop mild hypotension, while others become profoundly hypotensive. In some patients the only manifestations of gram-negative shock will be unexplained hypotension, unexplained oliguria, or unexplained tachypnea. When tachypnea and hypotension are the only signs, sepsis is frequently misdiagnosed as a pulmonary embolus. Some patients maintain good cerebral function up until the moment of death. Initially the white blood count may be decreased, but most patients develop a brisk leukocytosis. Persistent leukopenia is occasionally seen in *Pseudomonas* septicemia. Thrombocytopenia is also common. The blood gas determinations and blood pH are usually consistent with a respiratory alkalosis early in the course, and a metabolic acidosis appears later as lactate concentrations increase.

PATHOPHYSIOLOGY OF GRAM-NEGATIVE SEPTICEMIA

Although gram-negative bacteremia was recognized for many years, the concept of gram-negative septicemia was not defined as a syndrome until 1951. Since Waisbren's description over two decades ago, extensive investigation has been directed into the genesis of the clinical constellation of signs and symptoms known as endotoxic shock. At least three features appear to be interrelated in the syndrome: (1) immunochemical initiation and perpetuation, (2) disseminated intravascular coagulation with its concomitant effects, and (3) disruption of the microcirculation. The final common denominator is circulatory insufficiency secondary to inadequate tissue perfusion.

The semirigid gram-negative bacterial cell wall contains endotoxin, which is a lipopolysaccharide which appears to be liberated only during bacterial cell lysis and thereby initiates all or part of the clinical picture. Experimentally, intravenous endotoxin is characteristically found in the hepatic reticuloendothelial system (RES) as well as in the splenic macrophages, neutrophilic leukocytes, macrophages, and vascular endothelium. Rechallenge of the experimental animal or blockade of the RES with intravenous endotoxin produces the generalized Shwartzman reaction. Most of the data available on the effects of endotoxin derive from experimental animals, and often the doses employed are pharmacologic. In most of the animals studied the principal effects of endotoxin are hypotension, decreased cardiac output, decreased peripheral blood flow, decreased plasma volume, and oliguria. Autopsy studies vary according to species but show hemorrhagic congestion of lungs, liver, and kidneys. A consistent and striking feature is the extensive pooling of blood and hemorrhagic necrosis of the small bowel. How endotoxin mediates these effects is unclear; it may require intermediary plasma substances or may sensitize the vascular epithelium to the effects of epinephrine (see also p. 60). Many of these effects can be prevented by pretreating the experimental animal with adrenal corticosteroids.

One plasma factor that may be important as an intermediary is complement. A popular concept is that small amounts of antibody to endotoxin combine with endotoxin, complement is activated and, as it is consumed, biologically active intermediate products are generated. These products have effects similar to those described for endotoxin.

Another possible plasma factor that is activated by endotoxin is the kinin system. These are vasoactive polypeptides which, like the components of complement, can induce arteriolar dilation, vasoconstriction, increased capillary permeability, and hypotension. They are formed from the enzymatic action of kallikrein on an α-2 globulin (kininogen) and have recently received attention in endotoxemia. Kinins are activated in a cascade sequence much like the complement, clotting, and fibrinolysis systems. Hageman factor (XII) may initiate all three systems.

Another possible intermediary step is the release of lysosomal enzymes. The actions of many of the enzymes have properties consistent with the observed effects of endotoxin. These enzymes are not released in animals pretreated with cortisone.

The role of the microcirculation has received much attention in the pathogenesis of gram-negative septic shock. The microcirculation consists of arterioles, metarterioles, capillaries, venules, and precapillary and postcapillary sphincters. Most of the proposed intermediaries of the effects of endotoxin influence the microcirculatory blood flow, especially the kinins and lysosomal enzymes. Microcirculatory blood flow is also influenced by catecholamines, histamine, and serotonin. Lillehei and associates demonstrated in dogs in shock that the capillary beds of the splanchnic circulation become ischemic. This is due to precapillary and postcapillary constriction, presumably from catecholamine stimulation. Subsequently the precapillary sphincters relax, having become refractory to catecholamines because of local lactic acidosis. The postcapillary venous sphincters remain constricted since their physiologic pH range is lower. Consequently pooling in the capillary circuits ensues despite decreased venous return to a now compromised myocardium. This intravascular fluid loss results in a decreased cardiac output and progressively poorer perfusion of the general microcirculation. At some point in the sequence, the accumulated lactic acid resulting from anaerobic metabolisms begins to overwhelm the buffering capacities of the body and acidosis supervenes. As acidosis increases, the syndrome becomes progressively difficult to reverse, and death usually results.

BACTERIOLOGY

The bacteria responsible for gram-negative septicemia are part of the normal flora of the body. Their incidence in this syndrome reflects the normal aerobic gastrointestinal flora. The most commonly isolated organisms, in decreasing order of frequency, are *E. coli,* the *Enterobacter-Klebsiella* group, *Pseudomonas aeruginosa,* and *Proteus* species. *Bacteroides* and other anaerobes are being isolated with increasing frequency, and polymicrobial bacteremia occurs in 6 to 13% of patients. With certain predisposing conditions, the types of the bacteria change. For instance, in burns or leukemia *Pseudomonas* infection is more common; in postpartum or postabortal states or in gastrointestinal surgery *Bacteroides* infection is frequently found; and in chronic refractory urinary tract infection *Proteus* organisms may be responsible for gram-negative septicemia.

The most common source of gram-negative bacteria is the urinary tract, with the gastrointestinal tract second. Less commonly the respiratory tree is the portal of entry except when respiration is assisted or a tracheostomy is present. Other sources of bacteremia are indwelling polyethylene catheters, the reproductive system, and the integument; a few cases have been reported following transfusion. In certain instances the source of infection is inapparent; this is particularly true in leukemia, lymphoma, and in patients with otherwise compromised host defenses.

PREDISPOSING CONDITIONS

Gram-negative septicemia occurs in the very young, the elderly, and the debilitated. Those affected are usually hospitalized patients. Those diseases most commonly predisposing to sepsis are pyelonephritis, leukemia, lymphoma, other blood dyscrasias and malignancies, cirrhosis, and poorly controlled diabetes mellitus. Childbirth, septic abortion, burns, and trauma can also be included as predisposing causes.

Iatrogenic infection is a most important category. Genitourinary instrumentation, gastrointestinal and biliary surgery, immunosuppressive drugs, adrenal corticosteroids, irradiation therapy, prior antibiotic therapy, indwelling polyethylene catheters, urinary catheters, respirators, and tracheostomies all account for a significant number of infections.

The mechanisms for many of these natural and iatrogenic afflictions appear evident. Host defense mechanisms are impaired by leukemia, lymphoma, immunosuppressive drugs, corticosteroids, and irradiation. Antibiotics presumably select out the susceptible flora, allowing the antibiotic-resistant organisms to multiply. Surgery, instrumentation, and skin lesions destroy anatomic barriers. One possible mechanism for septicemia in cirrhosis is the presence of arteriovenous fistulas, which allow portal blood containing bacteria to bypass the liver.

TREATMENT

Since the pathophysiology is only partially understood and the hemodynamic measurements vary from patient to patient, one cannot be inflexible in his views on therapy. Rational therapy must be defined in light of a given patient and his particular response to infection. Prompt recognition and institution of therapy is of prime importance. Therapy can be divided arbitrarily into antibiotic therapy and therapy of shock.

Therapy of Shock

Therapy must be tailored to the clinical situation. Adequate tissue perfusion and an adequate plasma volume, hyperoxygenation of the blood, normal plasma pH, good urinary output, and a normal cardiac output are the goals of therapy. In order to make these judgments, the patient must be properly monitored with careful attention to intake and output values, central venous pressure determinations, and, where available, a Swan-Ganz catheter to help in evaluating left ventricular function. Frequent blood gas, pH, and lactate determinations are important. Good clinical observation, careful attention to the heart tones, including the pulmonary component of the second heart sound, and to the pulse contour, peripheral temperature and color, and mental function are often overlooked as important adjuncts in determining the choice of therapy.

Maintenance of a patent airway is a first consideration. The use of blood gas determinations may enable the clinician to anticipate the need for assisted ventilation. A decreasing Po_2 with a decreasing Pco_2 (inadequate hyperventilation) or with an increasing Pco_2 (poor ventilation) are indications for mechanical ventilation.

Central venous pressure monitoring is a good guide to volume replacement. Although its validity has been questioned since it appears that the central venous pressure reflects right heart competency and capacitance in the great veins, it remains a most useful bedside tool. Where available, a Swan-Ganz catheter is useful in assessment of left ventricular function.

Parenteral fluid administration is most important. Choices of intravenous fluids will vary with the individual. Synthetic extracellular fluid is a readily available physiologic replacement; it is made by mixing 750 ml. isotonic saline, 225 ml. 5% dextrose in water, and 25 ml. $NaHCO_3$ (3.75 gm. per 50 ml.) to provide 137 mEq. Na^+, 115 mEq. Cl^-, and 22.5 mEq. HCO_3^-. Lactate should be avoided since its metabolism in the liver is impaired in shock. Physiologic saline or 5% dextrose in saline may be suitable substitutes where colloids are not deemed necessary. Colloid expansion via low-molecular-weight dextrans (40,000 molecular weight range) has hypothetical advantages in that it may decrease red blood cell aggregation and prevent disseminated intravascular coagulation. Dextrans have been implicated in renal tubular obstruction and may increase intracellular and interstitial volume.

The use of adrenergic agents is controversial, but there is little evidence that they are of value. Alpha-adrenergic stimulators can produce intense vasoconstriction, which exacerbates the generalized vasoconstriction already occurring (see section Pathophysiology of Gram-Negative Septicemia, earlier in this chapter). Under these conditions they have little inotropic effect. Isoproterenol is a β-adrenergic stimulator with no α-adrenergic effects. It increases cardiac output, increases venous return to the heart, decreases peripheral vascular resistance, and increases renal blood flow. It may also decrease pulmonary vascular resistance and increase coronary perfusion. Isoproterenol is used when plasma expansion does not correct the hemodynamic abnormalities. Its use is usually followed by a lowering of the central venous pressure, an increase in urinary output, and a rise in the pulse pressure. Continued plasma expansion is necessary with isoproterenol to prevent hypotension secondary to vasodilation. A good guide is to keep the central venous pressure at about 16 cm. H_2O. Isoproterenol is administered by intravenous drip. The initial recommended concentration is 2.5 mg. in 500 ml. of 5% dextrose in water. The initial rate of infusion is 0.5 to 1 ml. per minute. The principal untoward effects are tachycardia, arrhythmias, and tachyphylaxis. The use of α-adrenergic blocking agents remains investigational, although it offers promise for the future.

Adrenal steroids are widely employed in the treatment of septic shock. The chief mechanism appears to be vasodilation. A dose of 2 gm. of hydrocortisone or its equivalent is administered over a three- to five-minute period. Increased oxygen consumption, a reduction in lactic acid levels, and an increase in urinary output are also observed. If used, adrenal steroids should be employed early in treatment in order that the vascular effects can be obtained. Corticosteroids are often given as a last resort, in which case they are of little or no value.

Antibiotic Therapy

The choice of an appropriate antibiotic should be based on the possible responsible bacteria and their probable sensitivity patterns.

Ampicillin is effective against most strains of *E. coli* and many *Klebsiella* and indole-negative *Proteus* species. The dosage recommended in gram-negative sepsis is 8 or more gm. per day administered intravenously in divided doses. The side effects are minimal except for the risk of penicillin allergy.

Carbenicillin has the same spectrum as ampicillin, but in addition it is effective against some ampicillin-resistant *E. coli, Enterobacter,* some indole-positive *Proteus* strains and *P. aeruginosa.* The dosage for gram-negative infections of the bloodstream is 8 or more gm. per day administered intravenously. In *Pseudomonas* infections the dosage is 30 to 40 gm. per day administered intravenously. One method is to administer the carbenicillin by continuous intravenous drip with concomitant probenecid therapy, 1 gm. by mouth every 6 hours. Many authorities opt for combined carbenicillin and gentamicin therapy in *Pseudomonas* infection. The latter is administered in maximum allowable intramuscular dosages. The side effects are minimal except for penicillin hypersensitivity.

Chloramphenicol shows a high degree of in vitro effectiveness against *E. coli, Enterobacter, Klebsiella,* and indole-negative *Proteus* species. Since it is a bacteriostatic agent, it should usually not be used in gram-negative septicemia. It is, however, the drug of choice for *Bacteroides* septicemia. Clindamycin in large intravenous doses may also be used in an anaerobic infection. Tetracycline has a spectrum similar to chloramphenicol but is less effective in general.

Polymyxins (Polymyxin B, colistin) are effective against *E.*

coli, Enterobacter, Klebsiella, and *Pseudomonas.* They are not effective against *Proteus* species. The use of the polymyxins in gram-negative septicemia is limited by their toxicity. In large doses they are neurotoxic and produce renal damage and, rarely, neuromuscular blockade. The drug is administered intramuscularly, 3 mg. per kilogram of body weight per day in two to three divided dosages.

Kanamycin is effective against the majority of strains responsible for gram-negative septicemia except *Pseudomonas* and *Bacteroides* infection. Its use is limited by eighth cranial nerve and renal toxicity. Some strains of gram-negative bacteria will be resistant to kanamycin and sensitive to gentamicin. Kanamycin is best administered intramuscularly in maximally allowable dosages (15 mg. per kilogram of body weight per day in two divided doses).

Gentamicin has the broadest antibacterial spectrum of any antibiotic against gram-negative bacteria. For this reason it is the drug of choice in undefined sepsis presumed to be due to a gram-negative bacillus. It is not effective against *Bacteroides* septicemia. Gentamicin is administered in maximal intramuscular dosages (5 mg. per kilogram of body weight per day in three divided doses). Its use is limited by renal and eighth cranial nerve toxicity.

Combined antibiotic therapy is widely employed in suspected gram-negative septicemia, and with good intent—to broaden the spectrum of coverage, to reduce toxicity of a given agent by allowing for reduction in dosage, to produce a synergistic bactericidal effect, and to reduce the emergence of resistant strains. Other possible and more practical reasons are the possibility of a gram-positive infection, a polymicrobial bacteremia, or an anaerobic infection. In the case in which *Pseudomonas* infection is likely, such as in leukemia, a combination of carbenicillin and gentamicin is acceptable. In undefined sepsis in which gram-positive infection is also likely, cephalothin or oxacillin may be added to gentamicin. In undefined sepsis in which anaerobic infection is suspected (postabortal, postpartum, or after gastrointestinal surgery), chloramphenicol is used. In undefined sepsis in which enterococcal infection is likely (following genitourinary instrumentation), ampicillin can be administered in addition to gentamicin.

PROGNOSIS

The mortality rate of gram-negative septicemia varies between 20 and 50%. Clearly it is higher in the elderly and in those with an illness that would normally be rapidly fatal (notably acute leukemia). The lower mortality rates are in young persons with postpartum or postabortal sepsis. The mortality rate is higher with *Pseudomonas* and polymicrobial septicemia than with other gram-negative bacteria; however, this is probably because most of the cases of *Pseudomonas* and polymicrobial septicemias occur in patients with severe illnesses. The fatality rate associated with gram-negative septicemia complicating surgical procedures or instrumentation is lower than that from septicemia not associated with operative procedures. The fatality rate for septicemia acquired outside the hospital is approximately one-half the rate for hospital-acquired septicemia.

PREVENTION

Since the urogenital tract is a major source of gram-negative bacteremia, every effort should be made to avoid unnecessary instrumentation or catheterization. When instrumentation is necessary, the urine should be rendered sterile prior to the procedure. When catheterization is necessary, every means should be taken to avoid infection: this means sterile gloves and aseptic technique, careful cleansing of the urethra, atraumatic technique, application of polyantibiotic cream at the urethral orifice, antibiotic rinse of the bladder, and connection of the catheter to closed drainage (see Chapter 6). Indwelling intravenous catheters should have limited indications for use. If they are necessary, the procedure should begin with an iodine and alcohol skin preparation, sterile gloves, a polyantibacterial cream, and a dressing. Indwelling polyethylene catheters should be removed after a maximum of three days. Similar careful attention should be paid to tracheostomy care and use of ventilation machines, and antibiotics, adrenal steroids, or immunosuppressive therapy should not be used except when there are well-defined indications.

REFERENCES

Christy, J. H. Pathophysiology of gram-negative shock. *Amer. Heart J.* 81:694, 1971.

Dietzman, R. H., Motsay, G. J., and Lillehei, R. C. Drugs in the treatment of shock. *Pharmacol. Physicians,* 1970 (August).

DuPont, H. L., and Spink, W. W. Infections due to gram-negative organisms: An analysis of 860 patients with bacteremia at the University of Minnesota Medical Center, 1958–1966. *Medicine* 48:307, 1969.

Gilbert, R. P. Mechanisms of hemodynamic effects of endotoxin. *Physiol. Rev.* 40:245, 1960.

Hemreck, A. S., and Thal, A. P. Mechanisms for the high circulatory requirements in sepsis and septic shock. *Ann. Surg.* 170:677, 1969.

Hodgin, U. G., and Sanford, J. P. Gram-negative rod bacteremia: An analysis of 100 patients. *Amer. J. Med.* 39:952, 1965.

Kardos, G. C. Isoproterenol in the treatment of shock due to bacteremia with gram-negative pathogens. *New Eng. J. Med.* 274:868, 1966.

McCabe, W. R., and Jackson, G. G. Gram-negative bacteremia: I. Etiology and ecology; II. Clinical, laboratory and therapeutic observations. *Arch. Intern. Med.* (Chicago) 110:847, 1962.

MacLean, L. D., Mulligan, W. G., McLean, A. P. H., and Duff, J. H. Patterns of septic shock in man—a detailed study of 56 patients. *Ann. Surg.* 166:543, 1967.

Martin, C. M., Cuomo, A. J., Geraghty, M. J., Zager, J. R., and Mandes, R. C. Gram-negative rod bacteremia. *J. Infect. Dis.* 119:506, 1969.

Sambhi, M. P., Weil, M. H., and Udhoj, V. N. Acute pharmacodynamic effects of glucocorticoids on cardiac output and related hemodynamic changes in normal patients and patients in shock. *Circulation* 31:523, 1965.

Siegel, J. H., Greenspan, M., and Del Guercio, L. R. M. Abnormal vascular tone, defective oxygen transport and myocardial failure in human septic shock. *Ann. Surg.* 165:504, 1967.

Waisbren, B. A. Bacteremia due to gram-negative bacteria other than *Salmonella. A.M.A. Arch. Int. Med.* 88:467, 1951.

Weil, M. H., Shubin, H., and Biddle, M. Shock caused by gram-negative microorganisms: Analysis of 169 cases. *Ann. Intern. Med.* 60:384, 1964.

Weinsten, L., and Klainer, A. S. Septic shock—pathogenesis and treatment. *New Eng. J. Med.* 274:950, 1966.

8 / BACTERIAL ENDOCARDITIS

Malcolm T. Foster, Jr., and
Hall E. Harrison

THE ADVENT of open-heart surgery, the discovery of new antibiotics, and the improvement of bacteriologic techniques have changed the recognition, the clinical course, and, in some instances, the prognosis of bacterial endocarditis. In addition to the penicillin-sensitive streptococci, other gram-positive organisms, gram-negative bacteria, and fungi are becoming increasingly prevalent as causes of endocarditis. The variety of causative organisms has increased the need for careful bacteriologic studies, including serum dilution techniques, to evaluate therapy. Open-heart surgery not only provides hope for people with residual damage from bacterial endocarditis but also has been advocated as an emergency measure when valvular destruction brings about hemodynamic deterioration. The prosthetic valve may also provide a site for infection, however, and thereby make a bacteriologic cure virtually impossible. In the following discussion we will emphasize the changes in the clinical management of this disease which have resulted from improvements in modern medicine.

Bacterial endocarditis might more appropriately be called *infective endovasculitis,* since the endothelial linings of blood vessels, as well as of the heart, can be involved and since organisms such as fungi and rickettsiae also may be incriminated as etiologic agents. This infective endovasculitis can be caused by a variety of agents, any one of which in a given patient may have an acute or subacute course. Although the disease is divided into acute and subacute bacterial endocarditis, this distinction is a clinical one and is irrespective of the organism involved.

Acute bacterial endocarditis usually implies infection with a more virulent organism such as *Staphylococcus aureus* or *Diplococcus pneumoniae* and a more rapidly progressive clinical course. It may occur on a previously damaged or on a normal heart valve. The course is usually more explosive in onset and the untreated disease is more rapidly progressive, with the outcome usually decided in a matter of days or weeks.

Subacute bacterial endocarditis has generally been associated with less virulent bacteria such as *Streptococcus* of the viridans group or other streptococci. The disease occurs on previously damaged valves, in certain types of congenital heart disease, or on prosthetic valves. It is characterized by an insidious onset and a protean course; if the disease remains untreated it extends over many weeks to months.

For purposes of discussion, bacterial endocarditis is classified as acute or subacute as described above. It is emphasized that these divisions are made on the basis of clinical presentation rather than the identity of the organism involved. Patients with bacterial endocarditis due to *S. aureus,* for example, may assume a subacute course, particularly when the infection is on the tricuspid valve, whereas some individuals with endocarditis caused by a streptococcus may present with a short history, marked toxemia, and severe congestive heart failure.

PATHOGENESIS

Bacterial endocarditis caused by pathogenic organisms such as *S. aureus* is most common when there is a source of persistent bacteremia, e.g., an indwelling polyethylene catheter, furuncles, or postoperative wound infection. With these agents either normal or abnormal valves may be affected. Less virulent organisms generally do not affect patients with normal hearts. Predisposing factors to infection by *Strep.* viridans species are congenital heart lesions (patent ductus arteriosus, ventricular septal defect, or congenital aortic stenosis), valves damaged by rheumatic fever, or prosthetic heart valves. In contradistinction to the bacterial endocarditis caused by virulent organisms, where persistent bacteremia is the rule, organisms considered nonpathogens may cause infection with a transient bacteremia secondary to even minor dental procedures such as cleansing of teeth, particularly when the gums are diseased.

The question of why damaged valves are subject to infection

by nonpathogens has not been answered, but Angrist and Oka [1] have proposed that platelet-fibrin clots form on damaged valve surfaces. These lesions are then inoculated at the time of bacteremia, the organisms escape normal host defense mechanisms since the thrombi are avascular, and further fibrin deposition aids in protecting the organisms. Proliferation of the infecting agent eventually results in invasion and destruction of the valve leaflet or valve ring. Although this hypothesis is attractive, it remains unproved.

Endocarditis usually occurs in areas subject to high pressure changes and on the valve surfaces subjected to the greatest trauma, i.e., the atrial side of the mitral valve, the ventricular side of the aortic valve, the wall of the right ventricle in a ventricular septal defect, the pulmonary artery side of the patent ductus arteriosus, and the venous side of an arteriovenous fistula. Bacterial endocarditis is not increased in low flow or low pressure lesions such as an atrial septal defect [2].

Once the infection is established, the following mechanisms may be invoked in the pathogenesis of the clinical manifestations.

1. A systemic infection will produce fever, tachycardia, anemia, and cachexia.
2. Valve destruction, perforation, rupture of chordae tendineae, and associated myocarditis will produce congestive heart failure and development of a murmur.
3. Emboli, both septic and sterile, explain many of the neurologic findings, splenomegaly, and acute vascular insufficiency in peripheral vessels. Vegetations from fungi are generally larger, and vessels such as the femoral artery may be occluded.
4. There is ample evidence now that antigen-antibody reaction may lead to hypersensitivity reactions or immune complex deposition and lesions in the skin, kidney, and central nervous system.

Underlying Disease

Congenital. Approximately 20% of all cases of bacterial endocarditis are associated with congenital heart disease. Bacterial endocarditis is a relatively common complication of those congenital lesions characterized by high flow or high pressure, such as patent ductus arteriosus and ventricular septal defect. In these lesions bacterial endocarditis will ultimately occur in 10 to 20% of all uncorrected cases. In the preantibiotic era, bacterial endocarditis accounted for approximately 20% of deaths associated with these lesions. Congenital lesions characterized by low flow and low pressure, such as an atrial septal defect, are rarely complicated by bacterial endocarditis. The bacteria and clinical manifestations associated with bacterial endocarditis in congenital heart disease do not differ appreciably from endocarditis associated with acquired valvular disease.

Acquired. In acquired valvular disease, bacterial endocarditis commonly involves the aortic and mitral valves, with only 5% of all cases involving the tricuspid or pulmonary valves. The most commonly identified underlying pathology is rheumatic heart disease, although bacterial endocarditis may complicate calcific aortic stenosis as well. The organisms involved are representative of endocarditis in general.

Following Open-Heart Surgery with Valve Replacement

Between 1 and 3% of patients who have open-heart surgery with valve replacement acquire bacterial endocarditis. This complication is more common following aortic valve replacement than mitral valve replacement and is more common with prosthetic valves than with a homograft. The bacteria involved are usually gram-positive cocci. *Staphylococcus epidermidis* (albus) is most common, followed by *S. aureus,* various streptococci, diphtheroids, pneumococci, and, rarely, other pathogens [3]. The onset may be insidious, and the clinical course may be variable. Diagnosis may be particularly difficult following open-heart surgery, as patients tend to be febrile and paravalvular leaks may be difficult to hear or differentiate from normal prosthetic valve murmurs. The classic manifestations of bacterial endocarditis are often absent. Sande and associates [4] compared 22 patients with prosthetic heart valves and sustained bacteremia in order to differentiate bacteremia with proved valvular infection from that not associated with endocarditis. The 11 patients with bacterial endocarditis tended to be infected at a more remote time; the median interval between operation and positive blood cultures was 60 days with a range of 10 to 360. The bacteria responsible tended to be gram-positive organisms, the course was inexorably progressive, antibiotic therapy was unsuccessful, and the mortality rate was 100%. The median time of bacteremia between operation and positive blood cultures in patients without endocarditis was 12 days, with a range of 3 to 85. The bacteria were usually gram-negative bacilli, and a favorable response to antimicrobial therapy occurred in over half the patients. Patients with endocarditis had no obvious source for bacteremia and generally manifested new or changing murmurs, whereas patients with bacteremia usually had an obvious source of bacteremia and did not develop changes in murmurs.

Drug Addiction

Infective endocarditis accounts for about 10% of all the infectious complications of intravenous drug use. This is two to three times higher than the incidence of bacterial endocarditis in nonaddicts with preexisting heart disease [5]. Moreover, the incidence of preexisting heart disease is only 27% in addicts compared to 80 to 90% of all other patients who develop endocarditis [6]. The following points warrant emphasis.

1. The valves most commonly infected are the aortic and the mitral valves. Normal valves are frequently attacked, and 24 to 44% of cases involve the tricuspid valve [5–7].
2. Approximately 33% of patients are infected with gram-negative bacteria or *Candida albicans*. Staphylococcal infections account for 25 to 47% of the cases [5, 7].
3. The bacterium responsible for tricuspid endocarditis in heroin addicts is nearly always *S. aureus* [5, 7].
4. Drug addicts with preexisting valvular disease and endocarditis appear to be infected with the same organisms as nonaddicts, with the infection localized predominantly on the aortic or mitral valve [5, 7].
5. The mortality rate in treated endocarditis in addicts is 70 to 75% [5, 7].

Tricuspid endocarditis is characterized by fever, septic pulmonary emboli, and bacteremia. Heart murmurs are usually absent. The peripheral manifestations of endocarditis may be present, depending on the length of illness prior to diagnosis [5, 6]. Staphylococcal tricuspid endocarditis may assume a deceptively benign course. Tricuspid endocarditis may be caused by many organisms, including *Pseudomonas* and *Candida,* and is frequently associated with treatment failure or relapse [5]. In these instances surgery may be employed.

Endocarditis Complicating Hemodialysis

Bacterial endocarditis is a recently described complication of intermittent hemodialysis. Goodman and associates reported 2 cases and mentioned 2 other possible ones [8]; King and associates added 2 [9]. Of the 4 reported cases, 2 were caused by α-hemolytic streptococci and 2 by enterococci. In none of the reported cases is it clear whether or not there was underlying heart disease. In 2, dental manipulation preceded occurrence. Endocarditis has previously been described in association with arteriovenous fistulas but always in association with an endarteritis [10].

BACTERIOLOGY

Approximately 50% of all cases of bacterial endocarditis are caused by *Streptococcus* species of the viridans group. Viridans streptococci are normally nonpathogenic bacteria which inhabit the upper respiratory tract; presumably they gain periodic access to the bloodstream during manipulation of the teeth, as happens in mastication, cleaning, or dental procedures. Other penicillin-sensitive streptococci, such as microaerophilic streptococci, may be similarly incriminated. These penicillin-sensitive streptococci are usually associated with a clinical picture of subacute bacterial endocarditis, and a damaged heart valve or congenital lesion is generally a prerequisite for infection. These infections are treated with penicillin, and the cure rate is the highest of all organisms, ranging to 95%. The vast majority of these α-hemolytic streptococci require a minimum inhibitory concentration (MIC) of less than 0.4 μg. per milliliter of penicillin. With some strains an increase in the bactericidal rate in vitro can be demonstrated by the addition of streptomycin, and some authors employ both drugs in treating streptococcal endocarditis.

Staphylococci account for 15 to 20% of all cases of bacterial endocarditis. These may be either *S. aureus* or *S. epidermidis*. Staphylococcal endocarditis is characteristically acute, but in certain instances it may be associated with a clinical picture of subacute disease. When the clinical course is acute, the bacterium is most likely to be a coagulase-positive *S. aureus* and a source for infection is usually evident (furuncles, indwelling polyethylene catheter, postoperative). In 50% of the patients the acute infection occurs on a normal heart valve, often the aortic valve. When the clinical course is subacute, the bacterium is more likely to be an *S. epidermidis*, a source for infection may not be evident, and the infection occurs on a damaged heart valve or prosthetic heart valve.

Staphylococcal tricuspid endocarditis may assume an acute or subacute course even though the organism is most often an *S. aureus*. Approximately 60% of the strains of *S. aureus* and 40% of the strains of *S. epidermidis* are resistant to penicillin; therefore the initial drug of choice is an isoxazolyl penicillin, cephalothin, or vancomycin. Penicillin G is the drug of choice in penicillin-sensitive strains. Cure rates range from 15 to 65%, according to the particular circumstances, with the survival in most series being between 25 and 45% [11].

Group D streptococci, commonly identified as enterococci, account for 10 to 15% of all cases of bacterial endocarditis. Enterococci are part of the normal gastrointestinal flora. Infection generally occurs on a preexisting heart lesion, but examples are recorded of enterococci attacking normal valves. The clinical picture is quite varied, but what distinguishes the enterococci most is their resistance to antibiotics. Enterococci are moderately insensitive to penicillin, requiring 1 to 3 μg. per milliliter to inhibit their growth in vitro (MIC) but ten to one hundred times that concentration to kill them (minimum bactericidal concentration, or MBC). The MIC and the MBC for ampicillin are approximately equal and are lower than penicillin, ranging from 0.12 to 2.5 μg. per milliliter. The clinical correlation is that penicillin alone frequently fails in enterococcal endocarditis, even in doses as high as 60 million units per day. Ampicillin has been used alone in a few patients with enterococcal endocarditis with some success [12–14].

Experiments by Jawetz and Gunnison [15] and Hunter [16] have demonstrated that the addition of streptomycin, which alone has no effect on enterococci, drastically lowered the MBC of penicillin and increased the rate of killing of enterococci. This was the first example of antibiotic synergism. Since this work was done, penicillin and streptomycin in combination have been used as the regimen of choice for enterococcal endocarditis [15, 16]. These original observations have been expanded to show that ampicillin or penicillin in combination with either streptomycin or kanamycin or gentamicin will usually produce the same synergistic effect. Occasional failures with the penicillin-streptomycin regimens have also shown lack of synergism in vitro. In these instances one of the other combinations is substituted, depending upon studies in vitro. Although the clinical response usually correlates well with the antibiotic sensitivities in vitro, infrequently there is a lack of correlation between therapeutic results and sensitivity tests. Nevertheless, these patients are cured often with penicillin and streptomycin when the tests in vitro failed to show this synergism [15–19].

An interesting observation, which may have a clinical counterpart, was made some years ago by Hunter [20]. When the phenomenon described in vitro with penicillin and streptomycin was performed in two separate tubes, one containing fibrin and the other not, the rate of bacterial killing was markedly inhibited by the presence of fibrin. The reason for this observation remains obscure.

DIAGNOSIS

The diagnosis of bacterial endocarditis is dependent upon a careful evaluation of the history, physical examination, and laboratory studies. The classic manifestations of bacterial endocarditis may be absent, or they may appear during the course of treatment; also many of the clinical findings have been described in other disease states and are not in any way specific for bacterial endocarditis. Osler's nodes have been described in systemic lupus erythematosus, splinter hemorrhages in scurvy and trichinosis, and petechiae in a host of conditions.

Some 80 to 90% of all cases of subacute bacterial endocarditis occur in patients with underlying heart disease. Though any prolonged febrile illness should be evaluated, its occurrence after minor surgical, dental, urologic, or gynecologic procedures in patients with heart disease should be carefully evaluated with blood cultures. In addition, recurrent febrile illnesses recalcitrant to therapy or with changes in cardiac compensation should lead the clinician to suspect bacterial endocarditis.

The clinical manifestations may be grouped into six categories: (1) nonspecific symptoms of infection, (2) metastatic infection, (3) cardiac manifestations, (4) embolic phenomena, (5) hypersensitivity reactions, and (6) neurologic manifestations.

Nonspecific Symptoms of Infection. In acute bacterial endocarditis the signs and symptoms are usually related to the septicemia, with chills and fever predominating. The onset is usually abrupt. In subacute bacterial endocarditis the onset is insidious and fever is moderate. Fever is the most consistent finding in bacterial endocarditis, although some patients with untreated subacute bacterial endocarditis will have afebrile periods that can last for days or weeks [21].

Chronic infection probably also accounts for the anemia, pallor, weight loss, and splenomegaly found in bacterial endocarditis. Surprisingly, a leukocytosis is found in only 50% of patients with subacute bacterial endocarditis. Histiocytes have been observed in endocarditis as well as other diseases; they are best identified in the first drop of blood obtained from pricking an ear lobe. In the absence of positive blood cultures, the finding of histiocytes can be helpful in establishing the diagnosis [22].

Metastatic Infection. Sepsis with virulent organisms such as *S. aureus* may lead to multiple abscesses in the lungs, brain, kidneys, skin, and joints. Meningitis may also occur.

Cardiac Manifestations. After fever, the most reliable sign in establishing the diagnosis is a heart murmur. Initially the murmur may not be evident, but as valvular tissue is destroyed, murmurs will be present in nearly all patients with valvular endocarditis. In ventricular septal defect or patent ductus arteriosus, there may be no changes in existing murmurs and new murmurs may not develop. Heart murmurs are likely to be absent in tricuspid endocarditis. Changing murmurs are very suggestive of bacterical endocarditis, and those which develop are due to valvular insufficiency. In general, lesions begin in the avascular sections of the valve leaflets, with subsequent valve perforation. Occasionally murmurs that are present during therapy disappear after successful therapy.

Embolic Phenomena. Both sterile and septic emboli may be seen at any time during therapy. Emboli to the central nervous system and kidneys are probably most common, but occlusion of the coronary arteries with myocardial infarction has been described. Mycotic aneurysms may develop, and the larger vegetations of fungal endocarditis may also obstruct major vessels such as the femoral artery.

Hypersensitivity Reactions. There is now increasing evidence that a variety of clinical manifestations related to the skin and kidneys are hypersensitivity reactions. Janeway's spots (small, painless, raised, purpuric lesions on the distal extremities), Osler's nodes (painful swellings in the fingertips or toes), splinter hemorrhages, and petechiae and Roth's spots (elliptical hemorrhagic areas in the retina) are now thought to be related to a vasculitis and not to embolization [23]. Renal lesions and positive rheumatoid factors are discussed in detail below.

Neurologic Manifestations. The neurologic manifestations merit special attention because they are common, may be the initial manifestation of the disease process, and are associated with an increased mortality. Their incidence has remained approximately the same since the introduction of antibiotics. Between 20 and 40% of patients with bacterial endocarditis demonstrate neuropsychiatric complications, and in one series the neurologic finding was the major presenting symptom.

The most common neuropsychiatric findings are cerebrovascular accidents and toxic encephalopathy (confusions, disorientation, delirium, hallucinations). Other manifestations include meningitis or encephalitis, brain abscesses, and less specific findings such as headaches, convulsions, cranial nerve involvement, mononeuritis, visual impairment, and dyskinesias [24, 25]. The mechanisms for most of these manifestations are not known. In cerebrovascular accidents emboli are incriminated, but other potential mechanisms are vasculitis, thrombosis, and rupture of a mycotic aneurysm. In the series reported by Jones et al. [25], cerebrovascular accidents were the most common neurologic manifestations of bacterial endocarditis; toxic encephalopathy was responsible for approximately 20% of the manifestations.

Rheumatoid Factor. Approximately 50% of patients with subacute bacterial endocarditis show some type of antigamma globulin factor as evidenced by a positive latex fixation test. Those patients most likely to have rheumatoid factor are characterized by elevated serum globulin levels and active subacute bacterial endocarditis of greater than six weeks' duration. The antigamma globulin factors produced during the course of subacute bacterial endocarditis fall rapidly after successful antimicrobial therapy.

Renal Lesions. Proteinuria, hematuria, red cell casts, and varying degrees of azotemia may be observed in endocarditis. Renal insufficiency and uremia was common in the preantibiotic era but has become rare in recent years except in prolonged or untreated cases. These manifestations have classically been ascribed to focal embolic glomerulonephritis. The responsible lesions are, in fact, not embolic and are usually diffuse. They represent an immune-complex glomerulonephritis with deposition of antigen-antibody complexes on the glomerular basement membrane. The progression of the renal lesions is usually reversed with appropriate antibiotic therapy. Immune-complex glomerulonephritis is more common in patients with abacteremic bacterial endocarditis. Embolism, infarction, and metastatic abscesses of the kidneys also occur in endocarditis but are considered to be of less importance [26].

Laboratory Diagnosis

Bacterial endocarditis is characterized by a persistent bacteremia; if pour plates are used the number of bacteria found will range from 10 to 100 per milliliter of blood, with half of the patients having less than 30 bacteria per milliliter. At least four sets of blood cultures should be obtained over a 24-hour period. The blood should be diluted by the media chosen by ten to one in order to dilute out serum factors which may inhibit growth. A variety of different media can be inoculated and cultured both aerobically and anaerobically. If the original set of cultures is negative, the laboratory should be instructed to hold them for two to three weeks, since some fastidious bacteria, particularly anaerobes, may require more time for growth.

TREATMENT OF BACTERIAL ENDOCARDITIS

Principles of Therapy

Therapy will vary with the causative agent and its antibiotic sensitivities. It also depends upon whether a foreign body is present or not, and in some instances surgery must be employed. Even in a given set of circumstances there may not be a consensus as to the route, dosage, or duration of therapy. Nevertheless, certain principles are applicable in the treatment of most cases of bacterial endocarditis and guide the physician in his selection of therapy.

1. The antibacterial regimen should be bactericidal for the infecting agent. Bacteriostatic antibiotics such as tetracycline, chloramphenicol, and erythromycin produce cures in only 30 to 40% of patients with infections by streptococci of the viridans group [27]. The bactericidal drugs such as penicillin are associated with much higher cure rates.

2. The antibiotic regimen chosen should produce a serum concentration which is bactericidal in vitro against the infecting organism at a dilution of one to eight or greater by either the tube or plate method. These studies, when combined with a broad empirical experience, will dictate proper antibiotic therapy. For instance, most streptococci require an MBC of less than 0.2 μg. per milliliter of penicillin, in which case the physician might use intramuscular penicillin; however, a strain requiring 1.0 μg. per milliliter MBC will require more aggressive therapy. In vitro sensitivity studies might show sensitivity to tetracycline or erythromycin, but there is a high failure rate with these bacteriostatic agents. Enterococci will usually be inhibited by 1 to 3 μg. per milliliter of penicillin, but combined chemotherapy with an aminoglycoside is usually necessary to eradicate the organism.

3. The duration of therapy has to be sufficient to sterilize the heart valves. Because of the malignant nature of this disease, therapy should be continued for a minimum of four weeks in sensitive streptococcal infections and six weeks in enterococcal and staphylococcal infections.

4. The route of therapy should be governed by the sensitivity of the bacterium and the pharmacodynamics of the antibiotic(s) chosen. Many patients with subacute bacterial endocarditis due to penicillin-sensitive streptococci have been successfully treated with phenoxymethyl penicillin taken orally; however, as a practical matter the physician cannot be assured that orally prescribed drugs are taken, and for that reason this route of administration should be reserved for exceptional circumstances.

Specific Pathogens

Streptococci of the viridans group and other penicillin-sensitive streptococci can be treated with 10 million units of crystalline penicillin G given intravenously over a 24-hour period for four weeks. Other regimens exist using a variety of penicillin preparations and routes of administration, but their use requires good laboratory facilities and cannot be recommended in general [28].

Staphylococcus aureus or epidermidis. Penicillin-sensitive staphylococci can be treated with 20 million units of crystalline penicillin G daily in divided doses administered intravenously every 6 hours for six weeks. Penicillin-resistant staphylococci can be treated with intravenous oxacillin or cloxacillin, 12 gm. per day in divided doses.

Enterococci. Enterococcal endocarditis should be treated with 20 million units of intravenous crystalline penicillin G per day combined with 1 gm. of streptomycin every 12 hours for six weeks. This regimen may fail and, with confirmation in vitro, ampicillin, 8 gm. per day, can be substituted for penicillin and combined with streptomycin, kanamycin, or gentamicin. Vancomycin, 1 gm. every 12 hours for six weeks, is a suitable alternate. Cephalothin is ineffective.

Gram-Negative Bacteria. The treatment of choice is determined by the antibiotic sensitivity data. Gentamicin in maximum intramuscular doses, with or without carbenicillin, is the drug of choice until the pathogen is identified and the sensitivities determined.

Treatment of Endocarditis with Negative Cultures

In the 10 to 15% of patients with negative blood cultures, the most commonly employed regimen has been that as outlined above for enterococcal endocarditis. In the case of treatment failure, this can be modified by the substitution of oxacillin or by doubling the penicillin dosage. A successful regimen, based on a clinical response, is then continued for six weeks.

Role of Surgery in Bacterial Endocarditis

Surgery can be employed in the case of failure of antibiotic therapy or for hemodynamic reasons such as perforation of a valve with intractable congestive heart failure or ruptured mitral chordae tendineae. Recent experience indicates that surgical replacement of an infected valve can take place after a few days of antibiotic therapy without any increased hazard of endocarditis involving the prosthesis, regardless of the organism or valve involved [29].

Alternate Antibiotic Therapy in Penicillin-Sensitive Patients

The choice of therapy in a patient allergic to penicillin is most difficult. The hazards of administration of the drug to an allergic individual are well known, but the treatment of endocarditis may, at times, require the use of this agent. If it is not possible to substitute an alternate drug, therapy with penicillin may be initiated with a scratch test (10,000 units per milliliter) or with the intradermal injection of 1 to 2 units. Although only about a third of persons with a history of penicillin allergy will actually exhibit a reaction when challenged, the usual measures for the treatment of anaphylaxis are mandatory. Generally it is advisable to try to rapidly desensitize the patient to penicillin and to use whatever pharmacologic means are necessary to control the allergic response. This often means the use of corticosteroids, antihistamines, and epinephrine. Alternate antibiotics for staphylococcal or streptococcal endocarditis are cephalothin or vancomycin. In enterococcal endocarditis, vancomycin is a suitable alternate [30, 31].

Assessment of Therapy

The clinical response to antibiotic therapy can be misleading. Some patients will appear to respond in a few days and yet have positive blood cultures. More commonly, patients are slow to improve and may even require weeks to become afebrile, yet their blood cultures will be sterile. Therefore, assessment of therapy must include follow-up blood cultures which are taken at three or more days after the initiation of therapy. During adequate therapy many patients will experience fever or embolic phenomena suggesting a bacterial relapse when, in fact, the infection is well controlled [32].

Relapse after Treatment

Relapse is handled in a similar manner as the original infection, but the duration of therapy is usually extended for an additional two weeks. Every effort is made to eliminate any cause of treatment failure.

Prophylactic Therapy

During certain procedures, patients at risk should receive prophylactic antibiotics. For tooth extractions, bronchoscopy, or tonsillectomy, 600,000 units of procaine penicillin may be given just prior to the procedure and repeated for the following two days. For cystostomy, transurethral resection, or normal vaginal delivery, 1,200,000 units of penicillin and 1.0 gm. of streptomycin are administered immediately prior to the procedure and every 12 hours for a total of three days. Prophylaxis is not generally recommended for cardiac catheterization. More radical approaches at prophylaxis, such as removing good teeth to prevent infections by streptococci of the viridans group, are of no value [33, 34].

In 1967 Doyle et al. [35] reported the results of observations on 1,762 children and adolescents receiving continuous antirheumatic prophylaxis. Sixteen cases of bacterial endocarditis occurred, making the risk of bacterial endocarditis to be 4.4 episodes per 1,000 patient years, a rate similar to that observed before prophylactic treatment was used. Although there was a slight increase in penicillin resistance among the viridans streptococci isolated from these patients, it was not clinically meaningful and there appeared to be no increased risk in patients receiving prophylactic penicillin.

REFERENCES

1. Angrist, A. A., and Oka, M. Pathogenesis of bacterial endocarditis. *J.A.M.A.* 183:249, 1963.
2. Rodbard, S. Blood velocity and endocarditis. *Circulation* 27:18, 1963.
3. Shafer, R. B., and Hall, W. H. Bacterial endocarditis following open heart surgery. *Amer. J. Cardiol.* 25:602, 1970.
4. Sande, M. A., Johnson, W. D., Jr., Hook, E. W., and Kaye, D. Sustained bacteremia in patients with prosthetic cardiac valves. *New Eng. J. Med.* 286:1067, 1972.
5. Andriole, V. T. Endocarditis in the drug user. *Conn. Med.* 34:327, 1970.
6. Conway, N. Endocarditis in heroin addicts. *Brit. Heart J.* 31:543, 1969.
7. Ramsey, R. A., Gunnar, R. M., and Tobin, J. R. Endocarditis in the drug addict. *Amer. J. Cardiol.* 25:608, 1970.
8. Goodman, J. S., Crews, H. D., Ginn, H. E., and Koenig, M. G. Bacterial endocarditis as a possible complication of chronic hemodialysis. *New Eng. J. Med.* 280:876, 1969.
9. King, L. H., Bradley, K. P., Shires, D. L., Donohue, J. P., and Glover, J. L. Bacterial endocarditis in chronic hemodialysis patients: A complication more common than previously suspected. *Surgery* 69:554, 1971.
10. Hook, E. W., Jr., Wainer, H. S., McGee, T. J., and Sellers, T. F., Jr. Acquired arterio-venous fistula with bacterial endocarditis and endarteritis. *J.A.M.A.* 164:1450, 1957.
11. Meade, R. H., III. Staphylococcal bacteremia and endocarditis. *Circulation* 19:440, 1959.
12. Mandell, G. L., Kaye, D., Levison, M. E., and Hook, E. W. Enterococcal endocarditis. *Arch. Intern. Med.* (Chicago) 125:258, 1970.
13. Beaty, H. N., Turck, M., and Petersdorf, R. M. Ampicillin in the treatment of enterococcal endocarditis. *Ann. Intern. Med.* 65:701, 1966.
14. Koenig, M. G., and Kaye, D. Enterococcal endocarditis—report of 19 cases with long-term follow-up data. *New Eng. J. Med.* 264:257, 1961.
15. Jawetz, E., and Gunnison, J. B. The determination of sensitivity to penicillin and streptomycin of enterococci and streptococci of the viridans groups. *J. Lab. Clin. Med.* 35:488, 1950.
16. Hunter, T. H. Speculations on the mechanism of cure of bacterial endocarditis. *J.A.M.A.* 144:524, 1950.
17. Watanakunakorn, C. Penicillin combined with gentamicin or streptomycin: Synergism against enterococci. *J. Infect. Dis.* 124:581, 1971.
18. Standiford, H. D., deMaine, J. B., and Kirby, W. M. M. Antibiotic synergism of enterococci—relation to inhibitory concentrations. *Arch. Intern. Med.* (Chicago) 126:255, 1970.
19. Tompsett, R., and Pizette, M. Enterococcal endocarditis—lack of cor-

relation between therapeutic results and antibiotic sensitivity tests. *Arch. Intern. Med.* 109:146, 1962.
20. Hunter, T. A. The treatment of some bacterial infections of the heart and pericardium. *Bull. N.Y. Acad. Med.* 28:214, 1952.
21. Kerr, A., Jr. *Subacute Bacterial Endocarditis.* R. L. Pullan (Ed.), Springfield, Ill.: Thomas, 1955.
22. Greenberg, M. S. Ear lobe histocytes as a clue to the diagnosis of subacute bacterial endocarditis. *Ann. Intern. Med.* 61:124, 1964.
23. Cordeiro, A., Costa, A., and Laginha, F. Immunologic phase of subacute bacterial endocarditis. A new concept and general considerations (editorial). *Amer. J. Cardiol.* 16:477, 1965.
24. Ziment, I. Nervous system complications in bacterial endocarditis. *Amer. J. Med.* 47:593, 1969.
25. Jones, H. R., Jr., Siekert, R. A., and Geraci, J. E. Neurological manifestations of bacterial endocarditis. *Ann. Intern. Med.* 71:21, 1969.
26. Gutman, R. A., Striker, G. E., Gilliland, B. C., and Cutler, R. E. The immune complex glomerulonephritis of bacterial endocarditis. *Medicine* 51:1, 1972.
27. Finland, M. Treatment of bacterial endocarditis. *New Eng. J. Med.* 250:419, 1954.
28. Quinn, E. L., and Cox, F. Bacterial Endocarditis: Based upon Experience with 203 Patients. In B. M. Kagan (Ed.), *Antimicrobial Therapy.* Philadelphia: Saunders, 1970.
29. Sarot, I. A., Weber, D., and Schechter, D. C. Cardiac surgery in active, primary infective endocarditis. *Chest* 57:58, 1970.
30. Raper, A. J., and Kemp, V. E. Use of steroids in penicillin-sensitive patients with bacterial endocarditis. *New Eng. J. Med.* 273:297, 1965.
31. Green, G. A., Peters, G. A., and Geraci, J. E. Treatment of bacterial endocarditis in patients with penicillin hypersensitivity. *Ann. Intern. Med.* 67:235, 1967.
32. Tompsett, R. Diagnosis and treatment of bacterial endocarditis. *D. M.*, September, 1964, p. 1.
33. Committee on Prevention of Rheumatic Fever and Bacterial Endocarditis. Prevention of bacterial endocarditis. *Circulation* 31:953, 1965.
34. Simon, D. S., and Goodwin, J. F. Should good teeth be extracted to prevent *Streptococcus* viridans endocarditis? *Lancet* 1:1207, 1971.
35. Doyle, E. F., Spagnulo, M., Taranta, A., Kuttner, A. G., Markowitz, M. The risk of bacterial endocarditis during antirheumatic prophylaxis. *J.A.M.A.* 201:807, 1967.

9 / MANAGEMENT OF TUBERCULOSIS IN THE COMMUNITY HOSPITAL

J. Joseph Marr

THE PAST TWENTY YEARS have wrought major changes in the management of pulmonary tuberculosis. These include improvements in diagnosis, therapy, and prevention both by the use of vaccines and sanitation, and by better understanding of the epidemiology of the disease. As a result of excellent public health work, the physician in this country is confronted with a disease which is somewhat different from that known to his predecessors. In areas where crowding is still prevalent and medical care substandard, such as in the inner cities of the United States, pulmonary tuberculosis still represents a public health problem; in the less densely populated areas, where nutrition and medical care are more adequate, tuberculosis has changed its clinical presentation.

There were about 35,000 new cases of active tuberculosis in the United States in 1971, with a new case rate of 17 per 100,000 population. Although the disease has declined in the world population as a whole, it is still an important cause of morbidity and mortality although the populations affected are somewhat different. This is most readily demonstrated by measuring skin-test reactivity to tuberculoprotein; the majority of the population under the age of 20 years is now nonreactive. As a result, the physician in the United States is more likely to see primary tuberculosis in the adolescent and young adult population. Hitherto this disease was a problem of the pediatrician, while the internist treated reactivation tuberculosis in adolescents and adults.

Newer antimicrobial agents are appearing and are being employed not only by those who deal primarily with tuberculosis but also by physicians generally as more tuberculosis is treated outside of the sanatorium. As our understanding of the pathogenesis and communicability of tuberculosis advances, increasing numbers of patients are being treated in the home or in community hospitals and the need for sanatoriums is declining.

A group of agents which is of variable clinical importance, depending on one's location in the country, is the atypical mycobacteria. *Mycobacterium kansasii* is not an uncommon pathogen and produces disease which is similar in every respect to typical tuberculosis caused by *M. tuberculosis.* The distinction between these two is important not only therapeutically but also from the public health standpoint, since the disease caused by the former appears not to be transmitted from person to person and isolation precautions are not necessary.

CLINICAL PRESENTATION

Early studies, both clinical and experimental, carried out by Rich and the more recent writings of Stead [1] have made it very clear that pulmonary tuberculosis undergoes the following sequence of events: the causative organism is inhaled, as a rule, from an individual with an active infection. These organisms are transmitted in fine-droplet nuclei and remain viable for a significant period of time despite desiccation. Contaminated food or drink is rarely dangerous. Most individuals infected with the organism do not develop disease but show evidence only of altered reactivity to tuberculoprotein; in others infection results in significant host injury. In this latter group the disease presents as primary pulmonary tuberculosis. The organisms produce a small initial lesion usually peripherally in the lung in the upper part of the lower lobe or in the lower portion of the upper lobe with involvement of the regional and perihilar lymph nodes. At some time during the spread of the disease from the periphery of the lung toward the hilum, hematogenous dissemination may occur, seeding the body with tubercle bacilli. Virtually all of these metastatic foci are eradicated by the now hypersensitive host defense mechanisms. The primary pulmonary lesion is contained generally by the bodily defenses, although if clinical disease does occur at this stage intensive chemotherapy can eradicate the organisms. The more usual picture is suppression or containment of the disease and calcification of the involved lymph nodes to produce the classic Ghon complex. The subsequent quiescent stage may last for the lifetime of the infected individual, or the disease may reactivate at a later time. The periods of peak reactivation are during the adolescent years, if the individual has been infected as a child, or in the late adult years during the sixth and seventh decades.

Although tuberculosis in adolescence has declined in recent years concurrent with the decrease in tuberculosis worldwide, it remains an important cause of death in this age group and poses special problems in diagnosis and treatment. Initial infection with the tubercle bacillus has become relatively more frequent in adolescents and young adults as the prevalence of tuberculosis has declined [2]. This phenomenon is especially noticed in economically privileged countries such as our own, where the annual tuberculin conversion rate rises rapidly from the age of 10 years on, concomitant with the period of more numerous social contacts outside the home. Many of these contacts are casual; Lloyd and McPherson found that 60% of adolescents with primary infection were unaware of the source of their infection [3]. In a more recent study of soldiers 17 to 20 years of age, Boyd noted that those with primary tuberculosis had a history of numerous possible contacts from the age of 16; in contrast, those with chronic pulmonary disease of the adult type usually showed a heavier family background of tuberculosis and known exposure to infection about four years earlier than the group with primary tuberculosis [4].

It is evident from the foregoing that the tuberculin skin test, long a useful tool for identifying those infected with tuberculosis in a population, is now of even more value. A positive reaction to mycobacterial purified protein derivative (PPD) in an adolescent or young adult may be taken as evidence for relatively recent infection, even in the absence of other clinical findings, and should be treated appropriately (see below). In some areas the prevalence of infection with *M. kansasii* may complicate the interpretation of a positive skin test. A reaction to PPD with greater than 10 mm. of induration at 48 hours is taken as evidence for infection with *M. tuberculosis.* Reactions of less than 5 mm. induration at 48 hours are interpreted as a negative response.

A recent report regarding the frequency of negative intermediate-strength tuberculin skin tests in persons with active tuberculosis has raised questions regarding the efficacy of some preparations of purified tuberculoprotein (PPD) [5]. There was a wide disparity of percent positive reactors using a commercial antigen and PPD-S (obtained from *M. tuberculosis*). The PPD stabilized with polysorbate 80 gave the greatest number of positive reactions. The major reason for false negatives and indeterminate responses to PPD appeared to be a loss of potency of the antigen due to adsorption. Experiments with radioactively labelled PPD have indicated that 72% of the radioactivity is adsorbed onto glass and 80% onto plastic in 24 hours. Polysorbate 80 is effective in preventing this adsorption. All of these observations suggest that loss of the antigen by adsorption to the vial and syringes is an important factor contributing to negative skin tests. Even with these precautions in skin testing, about 15 to 20% of individuals with active tuberculosis will not have a positive reaction. This is partially explained by extenuating clinical conditions such as old age, debility, or severe disease. The data from this report indicate that the most reliable antigen now available is the polysorbate 80-stabilized antigen.

An area of induration less than 10 mm. and greater than 5 mm. in diameter at 48 hours is indeterminate and may be a result of cross-reaction with the antigens of *M. kansasii* or group III organisms. The same is true for individuals reactive only to second-strength (250 units) PPD; many of these are infected with atypical mycobacteria and require differential testing [6]. In these instances repeat skin testing using the PPD-Y antigen obtained from *M. kansasii* may be of value. If the response to the latter antigen is greater than that to the PPD-S, then skin test reactivity is most likely due to infection with atypical mycobacteria. It is not necessary to treat persons with a positive skin test for *M. kansasii* unless there is corroborating clinical evidence of disease in the form of an infiltrate visible on a chest roentgenogram, cough, sputum production, isolation of the organisms from a patient's sputum, and so on.

Pulmonary disease due to infection with *M. kansasii* is usually slowly progressive and uncomplicated by the recovery of other pathogenic agents. However, chronic obstructive pulmonary disease frequently is observed in patients with these infections, which raises the question as to the role of nonspecific pulmonary pathology in favoring the retention and tissue invasion of an organism of borderline or diminished virulence. Of all the atypical mycobacteria, *M. kansasii* is most likely to show a favorable response to intensive antituberculosis chemotherapy. This is borne out in drug-susceptibility patterns, which reveal definite inhibition at higher concentrations of isoniazid (INH), and, to a lesser extent, of streptomycin and para-aminosalicylic acid (PASA) [7]. No clear-cut instance of human transmission of *M. kansasii* infection has been reported; therefore, it has been recommended that such patients not be subjected to the usual restrictions imposed on those with tuberculosis. Final judgment on the epidemiology of these infections must remain in abeyance due to the inadequacy of our current knowledge.

MANAGEMENT OF TUBERCULOSIS

The initial treatment for tuberculosis in the majority of cases should include a period of hospitalization. This provides an opportunity to obtain essential information pertinent to each patient and to permit the repetition of indicated procedures such as sputum and gastric cultures, liver function tests, roentgenograms, and pulmonary function tests. An essential advantage of an initial hospitalization is the opportunity which it provides to teach the patient about the transmission of tuberculosis and to firmly convince him of the importance of covering the nose and mouth when coughing or sneezing and to convey to him that cure of this disease will almost certainly be achieved. This facet of care of the tuberculosis patient—educating him about his disease—is many times overlooked and may be a common cause for therapeutic failure. If the patient does not understand that his disease is chronic and that he must take drugs for a long period, it is unreasonable for the physician to assume that the patient will continue to take medicines for the many months that are required for adequate chemotherapy.

The duration of initial hospitalization will require an individual judgment for each patient. Usually when a drug regimen has been found to be effective and when consistently negative sputum cultures have been confirmed, discharge from the hospital is in order. Such factors as home conditions, presence or absence of young children, anticipated reliability of continuing chemotherapy, and the general clinical status of the patient then become paramount in determining the final decision regarding discharge. In reliable patients whose follow-up is assured and in whom disease is only minimal, the initial hospitalization will be short and chemotherapy can be carried out at home. This necessarily demands that the physician be alert to the public health consequences and the necessity for repeated skin testing or prophylaxis of other persons living at the patient's home (see pp. 120–121).

The total extent and location of pulmonary tuberculosis is decided from examination of the chest roentgenogram. Although several views of the chest would be ideal for the establishment of the distribution and character of the disease, a single posteroanterior film may be sufficient. Pulmonary tuberculosis may be conveniently classified as:

Minimal. Minimal lesions include those that are of slight to moderate density but do not contain cavities. They may involve one or both lungs, but the total extent should not exceed the volume of lung which is present on one side above the second chondrosternal junction and the spine of the fourth cervical vertebra. This classification also applies to lesions that cannot be seen on the roentgenogram but which are associated with the confirmed finding of tubercle bacilli by culture.

Moderately Advanced. These lesions may be present in one or both lungs, and disseminated lesions of slight to moderate density may extend throughout the total volume of one lung or the equivalent in both lungs; total diameter of cavitation, if present, must be less than 4 cm.

Far Advanced. This term is used to describe lesions that are more extensive than those just named [8].

Currently there is little need to utilize drugs other than streptomycin, INH, or ethambutol for the treatment of patients who have had no prior chemotherapy. Cavitary disease, whether far advanced or moderately advanced, should be treated with a triple regimen. Minimal or moderately advanced noncavitary tuberculosis may be effectively treated with various double-drug regimens such as streptomycin-INH or INH-ethambutol. If there is any question as to the extent of the disease, triple therapy should be used. Virtually all tuberculosis seen in the community can be assumed to be caused by organisms which are sensitive to the above three drugs. If sputum or gastric cultures yield *M. kansasii,* then it may be necessary to obtain sensitivity determinations of the organism from the U.S. Public Health Service since this atypical mycobacterium is sometimes partially resistant to isoniazid.

A continuing study of drug resistance in tuberculosis in a U.S. Armed Forces veterans population by Hobby et al. [9] showed that in over 3,000 strains of *M. tuberculosis* recovered from nearly as many patients with newly diagnosed untreated pulmonary tuberculosis in 1965–69 there was no increase in resistance to INH as compared to comparable studies in 1962–63. Resistance to streptomycin appeared to be somewhat reduced from earlier studies. The incidence of strains resistant to three drugs, INH, streptomycin, and PASA, did not exceed 0.8% in 1968–69. Only 2 of 500 strains tested were resistant to rifampicin, and these were thought to have represented technical errors. These investigators concluded that after fifteen years of wide use there was no evidence to suggest that the prevalence of resistant organisms or of primary resistance to INH had increased. The value of the drug in the treatment of adult tuberculosis remains undiminished. In contrast, a study carried out at Kings County Medical Center in Brooklyn [10] on children during the years 1965–68 showed an increase in resistance to INH from 6 up to 10% as compared to the years 1961–64. There was a concomitant increase in resistance to streptomycin, from 3 to 10%, during this same time. The incidence of resistant strains in this community was relatively high. Although drug-resistant organisms remain infrequent among adults, they are apparently more common in children. This is compatible with the concept that childhood disease develops shortly after infection, whereas the disease in adults is often an endogenous exacerbation of an infection that may have occurred many years before. Infection with drug-resistant organisms in children is probably due to transmission of resistant strains from source cases in adults whose organisms become resistant as a result of failure of initial drug therapy.

Isoniazid. Isoniazid is very close to being an ideal drug for the treatment of tuberculosis. It is the least toxic of all available drugs, the most efficacious, and the least expensive. The most effective daily dosage of INH with the minimum number of side effects is 8 mg. per kilogram of body weight per day. This dosage was determined by studies on the reversion of tuberculin reactivity to nonreactivity in recently infected individuals using varying amounts of INH. In addition, 8 mg. per kilogram of body weight per day nullifies the rapid rate of acetylation of this drug, which is genetically determined and may be a problem at the lower dosage of 5 mg. per kilogram of body weight per day.

Isoniazid may be given in the traditional one-third of a total dose three times a day, but the highest serum levels are obtained by two divided doses or a single oral dose. On a regimen of 8 mg. per kilogram per day most persons will require about 600 mg. of the drug; this amount is probably best administered in two divided doses about 4 to 6 hours apart.

There have been several recent reports on INH-induced liver disease. The Center for Disease Control in Atlanta, Georgia, appointed an advisory committee to study this topic, and its report was published in July, 1971 [11]. The conclusions were that liver disease can occur in patients receiving isoniazid, although the risks of developing this complication are very small, varying from 0 to 10 cases per 1,000 patients on isoniazid per year; that the development of the disease is not predictable in any individual; and that INH-associated liver disease does not appear to occur in children. There were several areas of discussion in which general conclusions could not be developed: these included the degree of reversibility of the liver damage and the pathophysiology of INH-associated liver disease. The disease was placed in the category of "non-predictable, drug-induced hepatitis resembling viral hepatitis." It does not seem to be dose-dependent, nor are there any identifiable predisposing factors. The possibility remains that impurities in the drug may be the actual cause of the disease. The committee did recommend that screening procedures prior to the administration of INH should include investigation for the following.

1. History of prior reception of INH to exclude those who have had an adequate course of the drug
2. History of adverse reaction to INH
3. History of consuming other long-term medication, such as diphenylhydantoin, meprobamate, or hormones
4. History of symptoms or signs consistent with acute liver disease. Because INH-associated liver disease is viewed as an unpredictable hypersensitivity response, the committee thought that a history of past chronic liver disease (not associated with INH) was not necessarily a contraindication to initiation of INH preventive therapy. Routine monitoring for liver disease by laboratory tests was not recommended, since it was thought that these were not needed unless symptoms or signs of liver disease became evident

As with any drug, priorities must be considered in placing patients on preventive therapy. These priorities do not apply to individuals known to have tuberculosis; persons with known disease should be treated with INH unless one of the above contraindications is present. The following groups should receive consideration for the prophylactic administration of INH. They are listed in order of decreasing importance.

1. Household and other close associates of patients with active tuberculosis, both those who are tuberculin negative (especially children) and those who are tuberculin positive
2. Recent converters of any age. This may be defined as a change from negative reaction to a positive reaction or an increase of 6 mm. or more in a positive reaction
3. Tuberculin-positive individuals with pulmonary lesions of unknown etiology, i.e., compatible with tuberculosis but not sufficiently stable to be classified as inactive tuberculosis
4. Persons with inactive tuberculosis or residual fibrotic pulmonary disease presumed to have been tuberculous in origin
5. Individuals with a positive tuberculin reaction who have medical conditions such as leukemia, reticuloendothelial disease, gastrectomy, or are receiving immunosuppressive drugs

6. Positive tuberculin reactors under the age of 20
7. Other identified positive tuberculin reactors

Moulding [12] has analyzed the benefits of chemoprophylaxis of tuberculosis versus the risk and cost. After weighing the protective effect of prophylactic INH in terms of cases of tuberculosis prevented and comparing this with the cost to prevent one case in each of the categories, he was able to conclude that a strong recommendation could be made to give chemoprophylaxis to all children with primary tuberculosis and all persons with inactive tuberculosis. In persons in the intermediate situations, such as household contact and tuberculin-positive adolescents with normal chest films or tuberculin-positive adults with conditions that increase the risk of developing active tuberculosis (categories 3–6 in the list above), administration of the drug could be justified, but less well. In contrast, the rationale for giving INH to tuberculin-positive adults with normal chest roentgenograms could not be substantiated. Chemoprophylaxis of individuals who fall into category 7 in the list above may not be of value.

Streptomycin. Streptomycin may be given as 1 gm. intramuscularly daily for two to three months and then can be discontinued if a good therapeutic response has been observed. If not, the drug may be continued for an additional three to four months at a dosage of 1 gm. two to three times a week. Patients who have impaired renal function will require a different dosage schedule (Table 9-1).

TABLE 9-1 / Dose-Interval Modifications for Tuberculosis Patients with Impaired Renal Function

	Dose Interval as Based on Creatinine Clearance (ml./min.)			
Drug	100	80–50	50–10	$<$ 10
Streptomycin	12	24	24–72	72–96
Vancomycin	6	24–72	72–240	240
Kanamycin	8	24	24–72	72–96
INH	8	8	12	12–24
Ethambutol	24	24	24[a]	24[a]
PASA[b]	8	8	Not used	Not used
Rifampicin	8	8	8	8

[a] At creatinine clearances below 50 ml./min. use 15 mg./kg./day.
[b] At creatinine clearances below 50 ml./min. gastrointestinal toxicity is severe and acidosis is worsened.
NOTE: for more specific information regarding the use of this table, see Chapter 3.

Except for occasional instances of hypersensitivity, the major toxic effects of streptomycin are upon the eighth cranial nerve and the kidneys. Vertigo is generally not seen before the sixth or seventh week of therapy and will diminish when the drug is stopped. Hearing loss can occur in elderly patients or in those with renal disease. Vestibular and renal manifestations of streptomycin toxicity may disappear if the dose is reduced to 0.5 gm. daily. Hypersensitivity to streptomycin may be manifested as skin rash, fever, or malaise. In persons in whom renal failure is a major problem, it is reasonable to omit streptomycin from the therapeutic regimen and to substitute pyrazinamide or rifampicin.

Para-aminosalicylic Acid. This is the least potent of the initial therapeutic agents and has the greatest potential to produce hypersensitivity reactions and toxic manifestations. For these reasons it is gradually being replaced by ethambutol. Nevertheless, it is a valuable drug when used as an adjunct to INH therapy and usually can be maintained in most patients.

Gastrointestinal discomfort, varying from occasional diarrhea to severe nausea and vomiting with diarrhea, is the most common side effect. The side effects may often be controlled by the use of antispasmodics and sedatives and rarely require the cessation of PASA therapy. Gastrointestinal bleeding is occasionally a problem, and persons known to have active peptic ulcer disease or a previous history of such disease should be watched carefully. Hypersensitivity reactions are not infrequent and are manifested as fever, skin rashes, and occasionally a syndrome resembling infectious mononucleosis. The usual dose is 12 gm. per day in three divided doses.

Ethambutol. Because of the relative infrequency of unpleasant side effects, hypersensitivity, and severe toxicity, ethambutol is gradually replacing PASA as a primary treatment drug [13]. The recommended dosage is 15 to 25 mg. per kilogram of body weight per day. Some investigators favor using ethambutol at 25 mg. per kilogram for the first sixty days and then reducing the amount to 15 mg. per kilogram daily thereafter [14]. It is always used in conjunction with INH or INH-streptomycin in initial therapy.

The only significant toxic effect of the drug is retrobulbar neuritis with reduced visual acuity. The earliest change is a decreased ability to perceive the color green. It is important that each eye be checked separately, since unilateral retrobulbar neuritis has been reported. This complication resolves on withdrawal of the drug.

Pyrazinamide (PZA). This is a potent antituberculosis agent and is particularly valuable in multiple drug treatment regimens. The usual dose is 3 gm. per day using the following schedule: 1 gm. at 8:00

A.M. and 12:00 noon; 0.5 gm. at 10:00 A.M. and 4:00 P.M. The need to use this agent in the treatment of tuberculosis as seen in the community will be very rare, and because of its toxic effects its use probably should be restricted to hospitalized patients. Hepatotoxicity occurs in about 10% of those persons receiving the drug. All patients receiving PZA should be monitored for alterations in liver function, with serum glutamic oxaloacetic transaminase determinations being the most useful.

Rifampicin. This is a relatively new antibiotic that is extremely effective against tubercle bacilli. It has been used in England and Europe for several years but only recently has been approved for use in the United States. Its principal applicability is in the treatment of pulmonary tuberculosis, and it may be combined with INH, ethambutol, or streptomycin in initial therapy. Its major use to date has been in the retreatment of patients in whom the development of resistant organisms has prevented successful initial therapy [14]. *Mycobacterium tuberculosis* is highly susceptible to this drug, all organisms thus far tested having been inhibited by a concentration of 1 μg. per milliliter, a concentration easily achieved in the blood by the recommended dosage. The drug is usually administered at the rate of 600 mg. per day as a single dose or in two divided doses. Organisms resistant to INH and other antituberculosis drugs do not demonstrate cross-resistance to rifampicin [15].

Rifampicin toxicity is minimal and includes a few instances of thrombocytopenia and alterations in liver function tests. The latter side effects disappear when the drug is discontinued. In a series of 30 patients with far-advanced resistant pulmonary tuberculosis treated with this drug, no toxicity attributable to rifampicin was noted [14]. Rifampicin-resistant tubercle bacilli have been observed, so this agent should not be used alone.

Since the physician has at his disposal a number of very excellent chemotherapeutic agents for initial treatment of pulmonary tuberculosis, rifampicin should probably be withheld from the primary treatment regimen. Under certain conditions it will have a place in initial therapy; since it is excreted primarily by the liver it may be used in persons with renal failure who require treatment for tuberculosis (see Table 9-1), or it may be used in retreatment of individuals who have an infection with organisms known to be resistant to one or more of the other chemotherapeutic agents. Since the emergence of rifampicin-resistant tubercle bacilli has been observed, this drug should always be combined with another agent. An additional difficulty with the use of rifampicin is its cost; at current pricing rifampicin costs the patient about $1.00 per capsule.

Chemotherapy Summary. The available evidence justifies the conclusion that in far-advanced or moderately advanced pulmonary tuberculosis, initial therapy should include a triple-drug regimen. Streptomycin, INH, and ethambutol in combination provide the greatest effective coverage with the lowest toxicity. Streptomycin may be discontinued after 60 to 90 days, depending upon the rapidity with which the sputum culture become negative. If the sputum cultures are persistently positive, streptomycin may be continued up to 120 days at a reduced dosage. If the sputum cultures do not convert from positive to negative relatively rapidly, sensitivity testing should be done on the isolated organism to be certain that it is susceptible to the drugs being used. After streptomycin is discontinued, chemotherapy with INH and ethambutol should continue for the remainder of the first year. Therapy can then be continued with INH alone for an additional year, making the total duration of therapy two years. The available evidence now indicates that prolongation of a chemotherapeutic regimen to three years is probably no more effective than two years [16].

TREATMENT OF TUBERCULOSIS IN THE COMMUNITY HOSPITAL

The past two decades have yielded a more precise knowledge of the mechanisms of transmission and practical ways of disinfecting air. However, attitudes toward contagion and practices of handling of tuberculosis patients have not kept pace, and as a result, a rather elaborate system of precautions has been developed to protect persons who are in contact with an infected individual.

The tubercle bacillus is an organism that is readily killed by heat and sunshine or other sources of ultraviolet light. It is transmitted from person to person in droplet nuclei produced during coughing or sneezing by the infected patient. When air is exhaled from the lungs of the infected patient, small droplets of sputum are expelled as well. The larger particles fall to the ground very near the person who is coughing, while the smaller ones evaporate rapidly, leaving behind so-called droplet nuclei. Larger particles, even if inhaled by someone close to the patient, will be stopped in the nasal and upper respiratory passages and eliminated even though they may be laden with tubercle bacilli. Only the small-droplet nuclei containing individual tubercle bacilli can pass through the air passages to the terminal bronchioles and alveoli, where they settle out, survive, and multiply as infection becomes established. The available evidence suggests that tubercle bacilli on fomites—bed linen, furniture, floors, utensils—do not constitute a significant infection hazard. Most of these organisms die quickly as a result of drying, heat, or sunlight, and the simple measure of hand washing is efficacious in removing organisms which may have been acquired by contact. Therefore, breaking the chain of transmission of tubercle bacilli has two aspects: prevention of contamination of the air, and elimination of contamination once it has occurred.

Prevention of Contamination

Chemotherapy. The initial drug regimens outlined above ordinarily will reduce the cough and sputum of tuberculosis patients within a matter of days, and generally within a few weeks the excretion of viable tubercle bacilli is halted. The most effective measure for prevention of contamination is a good initial chemotherapeutic regimen. Occasionally a patient with drug-resistant organisms will constitute a special problem by continuing to excrete viable tubercle bacilli, but this will not usually be a problem in a community hospital.

Covering of Nose and Mouth. This is a precaution which should be taken by the patient whenever coughing, sneezing, laughing, raising sputum, and so forth. It is extremely effective in preventing aerosolized secretions from becoming airborne, thus breaking the transmission chain at its source. All raised sputum is expectorated into disposable tissues, placed in special containers, and burned or flushed into a sewage system.

Although gowns and masks have been the traditional means of preventing the spread of tuberculosis to hospital personnel, they are completely ineffective in preventing airborne infections and are not necessary. If anyone is to be masked, it should be the patient, and this is indicated only if he is unable or unwilling to cover his mouth when coughing.

Elimination of Contamination

The aim of decontamination is to remove from the air any tubercle bacilli excreted by the patient. These procedures should be applied to places where persons with unknown or unsuspected tuberculosis may be present, since it is these individuals who are most likely to transmit the disease. Because of the precautions taken in the care of persons with known tuberculosis, these individuals rarely transmit the disease, but emergency and admitting rooms of general hospitals and clinics and rooms used by patients until their chemotherapy has become effective are sites in which decontamination procedures should be followed.

Ventilation. The concentration of organisms in the air of a room and the likelihood of inhaling them is substantially reduced if the room is well ventilated. The simplest and most effective means for doing this is by opening windows or by using a small exhaust fan to remove air from the room to the outside.

Ultraviolet Light. The use of ultraviolet light is a valuable procedure for disinfection. Many studies have shown that the air of tuberculosis patients' rooms can be made noninfectious by irradiation. One or two rooms in any community hospital can be utilized for the care of tuberculosis patients by the placement of exhaust fans in a window and the installation of several ultraviolet bulbs mounted on the walls about six to eight feet above the floor so that only the upper half of the room is irradiated. As the air recirculates upward, most of the tubercle bacilli will be destroyed.

The efficacy of these simple measures of initial chemotherapy and adequate ventilation have been well demonstrated by studies in Veterans Administration hospitals [17]. The rate of conversion of the tuberculin test in these hospitals' personnel for the year 1963 was about 2.3%. At this rate the average time required for infection is about 43 years. This was achieved in spite of the fact that the Veterans Administration cares for large numbers of tuberculosis patients. Guidelines for the general hospital in the admission and care of tuberculosis patients have been published by the American Thoracic Society [18].

REFERENCES

1. Stead, W. W. Pathogenesis of a first episode of chronic pulmonary tuberculosis in man: recrudescence of residuals of the primary infection or exogenous reinfection? *Amer. Rev. Resp. Dis.* 95:729, 1967.
2. Smith, M. H. D. Tuberculosis in adolescents. *Clin. Pediat.* (Phila.) 6:9, 1967.
3. Lloyd, W. E., and McPherson, A. M. C. Pulmonary tuberculosis in young adults. *Brit. Med. J.* 2:1130, 1936.
4. Boyd, J. F. An attempt to determine the background to pulmonary tuberculosis in adolescent males. *Brit. J. Dis. Chest* 58:17, 1964.
5. Holden, M., Dubin, M. R., and Diamond, P. H. Frequency of negative intermediate-strength tuberculin sensitivity in patients with active tuberculosis. *New Eng. J. Med.* 285:1506, 1971.
6. Edwards, L. B. Current status of the tuberculin test. *Ann. N.Y. Acad. Sci.* 106:32, 1963.
7. Lester, W. Unclassified mycobacterial disease. *Ann. Rev. Med.* 17:351, 1966.
8. Diagnostic standards and classification of tuberculosis, National Tuberculosis and Respiratory Disease Association, New York, 1969, p. 69.
9. Hobby, G. L., Johnson, P. M., and Boytar-Papirnyik, V. Primary drug resistance: a continuing study of drug resistance in tuberculosis in a veteran population within the United States. *Amer. Rev. Resp. Dis.* 102:347, 1970.
10. Steiner, M., Steiner, P., and Schmidt, H. Primary drug-resistant tuberculosis in children. *Amer. Rev. Resp. Dis.* 102:75, 1970.

11. Center for Disease Control. *Morbid. and Mortal. Weekly Rep.* 20:231, 1971.
12. Moulding, T. Chemoprophylaxis of tuberculosis. When is the benefit worth the cost? *Ann. Intern. Med.* 74:761, 1971.
13. American Thoracic Society, Committee on Therapy. *Amer. Rev. Resp. Dis.* 98:320, 1968.
14. Vall-Spinoza, A., and Lester, T. W. Rifampin: characteristics and role in the chemotherapy of tuberculosis. *Ann. Intern. Med.* 74:758, 1971.
15. *Med. Lett. Drugs Ther.* 12:37, 1970.
16. Fox, W. Changing concepts in the chemotherapy of tuberculosis. *Amer. Rev. Resp. Dis.* 97:767, 1968.
17. Riley, R. L. Home vs. sanatorium care. *Amer. Rev. Resp. Dis.* 96:623, 1967.
18. American Thoracic Society, Committee for the Guidance of the Tuberculosis Program. *Amer. Rev. Resp. Dis.* 99:631, 1969.

10 / OPPORTUNISTIC INFECTIONS

Gerald Medoff and
George S. Kobayashi

Opportunistic infections are usually thought of as those caused by organisms not normally classified as pathogens which cause disease because of a derangement in host defense. In reality, any organism which infects a host accomplishes this by exploiting a defect in host resistance. Therefore, the most likely etiologic agent in any patient with an infection is the pathogen most prevalent in the environment at that particular time. On this basis, pneumococci, streptococci, staphylococci, salmonellae, shigellae, and coliform organisms are as likely to be the cause of infection in a patient with a defect in host resistance as they are in a normal individual. The differences between the two populations of patients lie mainly in their responses to infection and in the numbers of patients who are infected with "unusual" organisms. The host factors that are important in dealing with all types of infection are well described [1]. Usually more than one factor is involved, and their interaction is complex. The following will describe some of the more important infections and the host responses elicited by them.

HOST DEFENSES

There is a bacterial and fungal flora which is characteristic of various parts of the body [2]. The interaction of this indigenous flora with

Supported in part by grants from The John A. Hartford Foundation, Inc., and U.S. Public Health Service Grants AI 10622-01, AM 05611.

exogenously acquired pathogens has been demonstrated on skin and in the respiratory and gastrointestinal tracts [3]. Such antagonistic interactions probably enhance man's capacity to resist infection. An example of this is the interference with the growth of group A β-hemolytic streptococci which occurs when these bacteria are grown in the presence of *Streptococcus* of the viridans group, which is a normal inhabitant of the posterior pharynx of man [4]. The indigenous flora may be changed by a variety of factors, the most common being the use of antibiotics. Staphylococcal enteritis and oral thrush commonly occur under these conditions and probably result from the elimination of the protective normal flora [5]. Any physical or environmental alteration imposed on the host may also lead to a change in bacterial flora. For example, skin trauma such as burns or the use of occlusive dressings potentiates the growth of gram-negative bacteria and fungi such as *Pseudomonas aeruginosa* and *Mucor* species [6]. Even hospitalization alone, without any other predisposing factor, changes the usual bacterial makeup of the posterior pharynx and gastrointestinal tract [7]. These alterations are important not only because they eliminate the protective effect of bacterial interference but also because the newly populated bacteria themselves may act as a source of infection in the host.

The body has several anatomic barriers to infection. These include the skin, epiglottis, and cilia of the bronchial epithelium. Burns, trauma, and surgery destroy the function of the skin as a protective organ, whereas urinary and intravenous catheters and endotracheal intubation circumvent the other barriers. The recent epidemic of gram-negative bacteremia caused by contaminated intravenous solutions and the high incidence of urinary tract infection related to urinary catheters are examples of infections introduced when anatomic barriers are breached.

The most immediate host response to infection is the inflammatory reaction, and the polymorphonuclear leukocyte constitutes the essential factor in this response. Phagocytosis is the essence of this system and involves several steps. In the first, the bone marrow produces and mobilizes phagocytes in large numbers. Second, bacterial products or inflammatory mediators interact with serum factors, including complement, to attract phagocytes into injured or invaded areas by chemotaxis [8]. Third, factors in normal serum, particularly immunoglobulins, and the third component of complement, opsonify bacteria and thereby increase phagocytosis [9]. Fourth, the ingested bacteria are encased within phagocytic vesicles in the cytoplasm of the white blood cell. Fifth, cytoplasmic structures that contain hydrolytic enzymes fuse with the phagocytic vesicles and secrete their contents into the vesicle [10]. Diseases affecting phagocytosis and intracellular killing lead to an unusual quantity of infections with virulent and nonvirulent organisms. A decrease in the number of granulocytes can result from infiltration of the bone marrow with malignant cells, or bone marrow suppression from antimetabolites, irradiation, or other drugs. Defective chemotaxis, opsonification, ingestion, degranulation, or peroxidation occur in congenital disease or are acquired in diseases of the hematopoietic system or with use of various drugs [11].

If the phagocytes represent the first line of defense, then the monocytes and macrophages are the second [12]. Phagocytosis is also the function of this defensive system. Diseases involving the lymphoid or reticuloendothelial system, such as lymphoma, reticulum cell sarcoma, and solid tumors, or treatment with drugs such as steroids and antimetabolites compromise this defensive system and generally lead to infections caused by so-called intracellular pathogens. The response to intracellular infection which is mediated through monocytes and macrophages is termed *cellular immunity*. In addition to the mononuclear phagocytes, it is dependent on the presence of thymus-derived lymphocytes which constitute the greater part of the recirculating pool of small lymphocytes in the body. These cells can be specifically stimulated by contact with specific antigens. These stimulated lymphocytes then function in the following manner [13]:

1. They divide to form an expanded population of primed antigen-sensitive cells which make a major contribution to immunologic memory because of their long life span.
2. They may be "killer cells" which are cytotoxic for graft target cells.
3. They release a number of soluble factors which are chemotactic for monocytes and macrophages, inhibit their migration, and probably activate them. These factors are also mitogenic for other lymphocytes and increase vascular permeability. These characteristics form the basis for the phenomenon of specific cell-mediated immunity.
4. They may cooperate during the immune response to certain antigens by stimulating the nonthymus-derived or B lymphocytes to antibody production. The antibody produced by these lymphocytes is the basis of humoral immunity.

Primary specific immunodeficiency results from a failure to produce the effectors of the immune response (antibodies, sensitized lymphocytes). Antibody deficiency may be complete, with absence of IgG, IgM, and IgA, or it may be limited to one specific type [14].

Protection against infection with many respiratory and enteric viruses has better correlation with the presence of antibody in the mucous secretions than with humoral antibody [15]. The primary immunoglobulin in these secretions is secretory IgA. This antibody can neutralize virus and mediate lysis of some bacteria; however, it does not fix complement and is not opsonic. It may be that its biologic function is to sensitize the invading microorganisms to the bactericidal effect of lysozyme and proteolytic enzymes which are found in tears, saliva, nasal secretions, and gastrointestinal secretions. Hypercatabolic states, immune deficiency states due to exogenous causes such as x-rays or cytotoxic drugs, states associated with lymphopenia, neoplasm, or complement defects (C'_3, C'_5), and other congenital deficiency states are also included in the variable immunodeficiency category.

The relationship between immune deficiency and infection is complex, but generally those patients with deficiencies in antibody production tend to have multiple bacterial infections, usually with the usual pathogens. Patients with defects in cellular immunity tend to have intracellular infections (tuberculosis, fungi, *Salmonella, Listeria*). The patients with combined deficiency states are most severely affected and are troubled by infections of all types [11].

ETIOLOGIC AGENTS IN OPPORTUNISTIC INFECTIONS

Although bacteria are the most common opportunists affecting every type of compromised host, it has become clear that certain disease states are associated with an increased incidence of infection with very specific pathogens. The occurrence of *Salmonella* infections in patients with sickle cell disease [16], pneumococcal peritonitis in patients with the nephrotic syndrome [17], *Pseudomonas* pneumonia in patients on respirators [18], herpes zoster in patients with lymphoma [19], and rhinocerebral mucormycosis in patients with diabetic acidosis [20] are all examples of this association. Although virtually any organism can cause disease in the host rendered susceptible by some breakdown in normal defense mechanisms, the discussion following will be limited to a number of representative organisms.

Bacteria

Systemic or pulmonic infections caused by gram-negative bacilli account for the majority of deaths in leukemia and lymphoma [21]. *Pseudomonas* species are responsible for almost half of these infections. Other organisms frequently identified with overwhelming infections in this group are the gram-negative coliform organisms, *Klebsiella-*

Enterobacter-Serratia group, *Proteus, Bacteroides, Salmonella,* and the gram-positive organisms including streptococci, clostridia (with and without gas production), and, more rarely, *Listeria monocytogenes.* Of more serious consequence are episodes of septicemia caused by organisms of more than one type. In most cases, the infecting organism is disseminated from the patient's endogenous flora, which is itself influenced by the environment, and by other factors such as whether or not the patient has been treated with antibiotics [22]. Therefore, in devising empirical antibiotic therapy for the infected patient before culture results are available, consideration must be given to whether the patient became infected at home or in the hospital and whether antibiotics were being used at the time of onset of infection.

Fungi

As discussed previously, the debilitated patient is particularly susceptible to infections caused by fungi [23]. For the most part, these individuals are compromised by underlying diseases that affect the cells which mediate cellular and humoral immunity. Some of these underlying situations are a result of metabolic problems, others a result of genetic disorders, and still others of neoplastic origin. Agents and treatments which have an adverse effect on the immune response also place the patient receiving such treatment in a vulnerable position in regard to infection by opportunistic fungi.

Fungal infections may be divided into two distinct groups based on the morphology of the infecting agent [24]: the yeasts, which are primarily unicellular, and the molds, which are filamentous. The most common yeastlike fungus implicated in opportunistic infection is *Candida albicans.* This infection, unlike most other fungus infections, is endogenous in origin. Because *C. albicans* is part of the normal flora of the gastrointestinal tract and frequently inhabits mucous membranes, it is difficult to assess its significance when cultured from these areas. Other species of *Candida* have also been implicated in disease. Yeasts other than *Candida,* such as *Torulopsis glabrata,* are commonly isolated from the pulmonary and gastrointestinal tract and cause infections. As with *Candida,* it is often difficult to evaluate the significance of positive cultures.

Unlike the yeasts belonging to the genera *Candida* and *Torulopsis, Cryptococcus neoformans* is not part of the endogenous flora of man [25]. It occurs widely in nature as a soil saprophyte, particularly soil contaminated with pigeon excreta. Positive cultures of *C. neoformans* must always be considered significant.

The fungi which exist in filamentous form in tissue and in culture comprise the greater number of genera. Phycomycosis is an inclusive term which delineates disease caused by fungi belonging to the taxonomic class Phycomycetes. These fungi are primitive and are characterized morphologically by their relative lack of septation in the hyphae. Several genera have been implicated in disease. These are *Absidia, Mucor, Rhizopus,* and *Mortierella* [24]. Disease caused by these organisms is often a fulminating infection of the orbital sinuses which extends into the central nervous system. Pulmonary and cutaneous diseases are seen less frequently.

Members of the genus *Aspergillus* may be implicated also as a cause of infection in the compromised host. The most common clinical manifestation of aspergillosis is a lung infection, in which the fungus may exist either as the primary agent or as a secondary invader. The species most frequently isolated is *A. fumigatus,* but *A. flavus* and other species have been isolated from clinical material. The diagnosis is made by the demonstration of septate fungal filaments in pathologic specimens along with the isolation of the fungus in culture. Other filamentous fungi have caused clinical infections, but in general such infections are rare.

Viruses

Three of the four viruses which most frequently cause severe disseminated disease in the compromised host are DNA viruses that normally live in a symbiotic relationship with mammalian cells [27]. Destruction of the host cells or impairment of their function by cytotoxic agents, irradiation, and other therapeutic modalities or by underlying disease such as certain malignancies disturb this relationship and activate the viruses. The best example of this is herpes zoster, which characteristically remains latent for years until activated by one of the above. Similarly herpes simplex, aided by a defective host immunity, can cause severe necrotizing local lesions of mucous membranes or can disseminate rapidly to cause widespread fulminant infection [28]. The other DNA virus, cytomegalovirus, causes overt disease almost exclusively during states of inadequate immunologic responsiveness. Pulmonary involvement appears to be more common in adults, but hepatitis and kidney and bowel involvement, as well as lymphatic involvement, also occur [29].

Vaccinia is an RNA virus which causes a number of serious complications when individuals with disturbances of the cutaneous anatomic barrier to infection (eczema) or defects of humoral or cellular immunity are vaccinated [30]. The commonest complications of smallpox vaccination are generalized vaccinia and eczema vaccinatum.

Generalized Vaccinia. This potentially serious complication develops between the seventh and fourteenth day following vaccination. A generalized eruption develops with crops of lesions simulating a primary vaccination. Healing without scarring takes place rapidly, being completed at the same time as the primary vaccine lesion. The mortality rate in patients without eczema is quite low.

Eczema Vaccinatum. This potentially fatal complication of vaccinia develops in infants with eczema or adults with a variety of other skin diseases who have been either vaccinated or exposed to an active case of vaccinia. The disease is characterized by high fever, severe toxicity, and an extensive vesicular and pustular eruption chiefly confined to the area of dermatitis.

Vaccinia Gangrenosa. A usually fatal complication which is fortunately rare. The initial vaccinal lesion fails to heal and enlarges to involve greater areas of adjacent skin, often over a period of months. This serious complication has been observed in infants with immunologic disorders affecting the usual response to vaccination. It is also likely to occur in patients with immunologic defects caused by malignant diseases of the lymphatic system. These complications of smallpox vaccination illustrate the point that live vaccines should not be given to individuals with defective immune systems.

PROTOZOA

Surveys have shown that *Toxoplasma gondii* is present in approximately 30–50% of the population, yet toxoplasmosis is a rare disease in otherwise normal individuals [31]. The congenital form closely resembles neonatal rubella. Infections in older age groups are generally subclinical but can present with a typhoidlike syndrome or mimic infectious mononucleosis with fever, adenopathy, and atypical lymphocytes [30]. It is also a cause of posterior uveitis and may cause encephalitis or myocarditis. All of these syndromes, particularly the systemic ones with fever, have been observed as a complication of malignant disease. Because cell-mediated immunity seems particularly important in the defense against toxoplasma infection, diseases such as Hodgkin's disease, which are characterized by impairment of cell-mediated immunity, are more often complicated by toxoplasmosis.

Another opportunistic pathogen thought to be a protozoan is *Pneumocystis carinii* [32]. Following World War II, *P. carinii* pneumonia, originally designated interstitial plasma cell pneumonia, appeared as an epidemic disease of debilitated or premature infants in central Europe. With the exception of one reported outbreak, *P. carinii* pneumonia in the United States has been sporadic, occurring mainly in patients with malignancies, in persons receiving immunosuppressive or cytotoxic therapy, and in children with primary immune deficiency diseases. In the immunosuppressed patient it produces a rapidly progressive pneumonia. One study from the National Cancer Institute showed that in about 40% of patients with diffuse interstitial pneumonia, *Pneumocystis* was the etiologic agent [21].

DIAGNOSIS

Specific treatment regimens are available for most opportunistic pathogens, but the drugs themselves are usually quite toxic. By treating empirically with so-called umbrella therapy the hazards can be compounded and the opportunity to use appropriate therapy lost; therefore in most cases it is critical to obtain a definitive etiologic diagnosis.

In most patients who are prone to opportunistic infection, the presence of fever may not be diagnostic of infection but secondary to the underlying disease, for example, organ rejection in the transplant recipient or exacerbation of disease in the patient with leukemia. For this reason, the first question in evaluating these patients is whether or not they have infection. If the patient is seriously ill, treatment should be immediate and empiric after appropriate cultures have been taken. If not, it is reasonable to proceed with a diagnostic evaluation and observation.

Cultures and direct microscopical examination of clinical material are the most important tools of diagnosis in any suspected infection. Sputum, urine, stool, and blood cultures are monitored in any patient with compromised host defenses even before clinical infection becomes evident. A spinal fluid examination should be performed on any such patient with central nervous system findings or a persistent unexplained fever. The specimens obtained are cultured for the tubercle bacillus and for bacteria both anaerobically and aerobically. Sputum and spinal fluid are stained for acid-fast bacilli and bacteria. Sputum may also be stained with methenamine silver to detect *P. carinii,* although the yield from this procedure is quite low. India ink preparations of spinal fluid can be done to look for cryptococci. Serological tests for the presence of cryptococcal antigen or antibody to cryptococci in blood or spinal fluid are available and can be quite helpful in the diagnosis of this infection [33].

Direct microscopical examination of the clinical specimen may provide useful information in the diagnosis of a mycotic infection. The method of treating clinical material for direct examination will vary depending on its source. In general, solid pieces of tissues must be treated with a clearing agent, such as 10% potassium hydroxide, before they are examined microscopically. Fluids such as urine and spinal fluid should be examined microscopically, the latter with India ink, and the remainder of the specimen seeded onto a suitable culture medium. One should employ at least two types of media, one with and one without antibiotics. All cultures should be held for four weeks before being discarded.

Other accessible sources of material for culture and histologic examination are the bone marrow and liver. The presence or suspicion of a pulmonary infection in a patient unable to produce sputum is an indication for transtracheal aspiration to obtain material for culture [34]. If this is unsuccessful, brush biopsy or closed or open lung biopsy should be considered.

In addition to cultures, serologic tests can be useful in diagnosing a variety of infections. Serologic tests for agglutinating and complement-fixing antibody against *Histoplasma capsulatum, Blastomyces dermatitidis,* and *Coccidioides immitis* are available. Recently, tests for both precipitin and agglutinating antibodies to *Candida* and *Aspergillus* have been developed and are currently being evaluated for their clinical importance [35]. Skin tests for histoplasmosis, blastomycosis, and coccidioidomycosis are available but should be applied only after the serologic titer [36]. The tuberculin skin test, using both typical and atypical antigens, still remains an important diagnostic test. However, the compromised patient is often anergic as a result of either the underlying disease or of treatment [37]. Anergy can be documented by skin testing the patient for reactivity to mumps and *Candida* antigens and also by stimulation of skin reactivity to dinitrochlorobenzene. This can give important information about the immunologic competence of the individual.

Generally, viral infections are diagnosed retrospectively by a rise in serologic titers, but varicella-zoster, herpes simplex, and vaccinia viruses can be grown from vesicular lesions. The herpes group can also be differentiated from vaccinia by the presence of multinucleated giant cells on Giemsa stain of scrapings from the vesicular lesions (Tzank test) [38]. The characteristic owl-eye cells can be seen in the urine or in tissue in cytomegalovirus infection [39].

Pneumocystis carinii infection is diagnosed histologically from lung tissue. The organism cannot be cultured, and the serologic test is unreliable.

Taxoplasma gondii can be isolated from tissue or bone marrow and seen histologically. The organism can also be recovered from mice injected with tissue extracts containing the protozoan. The infection is most commonly diagnosed serologically using the Sabin-Feldman dye titer or indirect fluorescence. The latter test has been adopted for the determination of IgM *Toxoplasma* antibody by sucrose gradient ultracentrifugation or by reductive cleavage of IgM using 2-mercaptoethanol. The presence of IgM antibody is suggestive of recent infection [31].

THERAPY

A vigorous diagnostic effort in patients ill with an opportunistic infection is quite justified, since in most cases effective therapy is available. For bacterial infections, appropriate antibiotics should be chosen based on sensitivity testing of the organisms isolated. The use of carbenicillin and gentamicin to treat *Pseudomonas* infection has considerably improved survival of patients with this infection [40]. When treatment must be initiated before culture reports are available and there are no clues as to the etiologic organism, the use of a penicillinase-resistant penicillin and gentamicin is recommended. If one suspects *Bacteroides* infection because of symptoms or signs referable to the bowel, chloramphenicol is the drug of choice [41]. The higher bacteria *Actinomyces israelii* [42] and *Nocardia asteroides* [43] are treated with penicillin and sulfa, respectively. These last two infections require treatment for as long as six months.

Amphotericin B is the most effective drug for the treatment of fungus infections [44]. 5-Fluorocytosine is also available for use in *Candida* and cryptococcal infections, but thus far the high percentage of resistant *Candida* strains and the development of resistance in cryptococci has limited its usefulness [45]. Recently amphotericin B in combination with 5-fluorocytosine has been shown to be synergistic against yeast [46].

Cytosine arabinoside, adenosine arabinoside, and iododeoxyuridine have been used to treat cytomegalovirus, herpes simplex, and varicella-zoster infections with mixed results [47]. Our own experience with these drugs has been disappointing, but more patients will have to be treated before a final conclusion is reached. Other antiviral therapeutic regimens are mainly prophylactic, such as the use of zoster-immune globulin to prevent chickenpox [48] and amantidine to prevent influenza [49]. Vaccinia-immune globulin [50] and Marboran [51] have been useful to prevent the progression of eczema vaccinatum or vaccinia gangrenosa.

Toxoplasma infection is treated with pyrimethamine and sulfadiazine [52] in combination. This regimen is also useful against *Pneumocystis* [53]. The drug of choice in the latter infection, however, is pentamidine isethionate [54].

Because many patients lack specific components of host immunity, the appropriate antibiotics are frequently not sufficient to deal with the infection. In these circumstances experimental approaches to the therapy of established infection have been used. Granulocyte transfusions have been given to patients with aplastic anemia [55]. Transfer factor, the material extracted from the lymphocytes of healthy individuals, has been given to patients with defective cellular immunity [56], and gamma globulin has been given to patients who lack humoral resistance [57]. All of these procedures are experimental but are worth consideration in desperate situations.

An important consideration with regard to opportunistic infection is prevention. Specific immune globulins, such as zoster-immune globulin, have been shown to be effective in preventing or ameliorating the clinical manifestations of certain viral infections [48]. Isoniazid has been used prophylactically in patients with a risk of developing active tuberculosis. Some investigators have tried special isolation units, of which the most successful has been the laminar airflow room [58]. These patients are also given broad-spectrum antibiotics prophylactically. These studies are difficult to evaluate, and their great cost precludes general use, but preliminary trials have suggested some patient benefit.

REFERENCES

1. Klainer, A. S., and Beisel, W. R. Opportunistic infection: A review. *Amer. J. Med. Sci.* 258:431, 1969.
2. Marples, M. J. *The Ecology of the Human Skin.* Springfield, Ill.: Thomas, 1965.
3. Shinefield, H. R., Ribble, J. C., Eichenwald, H. F., Boris, M., and Sutherland, J. M. Bacterial Interference. In H. I. Maibach and G. Hildick-Smith (Eds.), *Skin Bacteria and Their Role in Infection.* New York: Blakiston Div., McGraw-Hill, 1965. Chap. 17.
4. Sanders, E. Bacterial interference: I. Its occurrence among the respiratory tract flora and characterization of inhibition of group A streptococci by viridans streptococci. *J. Infect. Dis.* 120:698, 1969.
5. McCoy, E. Changes in the host flora induced by chemotherapeutic agents. *Ann. Rev. Microbiol.* 8:257, 1954.
6. Swartz, M. N., and Weinberg, A. N. Bacterial Diseases with Cutaneous Involvement. In T. B. Fitzpatrick, K. A. Arndt, W. H. Clark, A. Z. Eisen, E. J. Van Scott, and J. H. Vaughn (Eds.), *Dermatology in General Medicine.* New York: Blakiston Div., McGraw-Hill, 1971. Chap. 23, pp. 1679–1845.
7. Johanson, W. G., Pierce, A. K., and Sanford, J. P. Changing pharyngeal bacterial flora of hospitalized patients. *New Eng. J. Med.* 281:1137, 1969.
8. Muller-Eberhard, H. J. Chemistry and reaction mechanism of complement. *Advances Immun.* 8:2, 1968.
9. Johnson, R. B., Jr., Klemperer, M. R., and Alper, C. A. The enhance-

ment of bacterial phagocytosis by serum: The role of complement components and two cofactors. *J. Exp. Med.* 129:1275, 1969.
10. Bachner, R. L., Karnovsky, M. J., and Karnovsky, M. L. Degranulation of leukocytes in chronic granulomatous disease. *J. Clin. Invest.* 48:187, 1969.
11. Dossett, J. H. Microbial defenses of the child and man. *Pediat. Clin. N. Amer.* 19:355, 1972.
12. Mackaness, G. B. The monocyte in cellular immunity. *Seminars Hemat.* 8:172, 1970.
13. Pearsall, N. N., and Weiser, R. S. *The Macrophage.* Philadelphia: Lea & Febiger, 1970.
14. Rosen, F. S., and Janeway, C. A. The antibody deficiency syndrome. *New Eng. J. Med.* 275:709, 769, 1966.
15. Orga, P. L., and Karzon, A. T. The role of immunoglobulins in the mechanisms of mucosal immunity to virus infection. *Pediat. Clin. N. Amer.* 17:385, 1970.
16. Silver, H. K., Simon, J. L., and Clement, D. H. *Salmonella* osteomyelitis and abnormal hemoglobin disease. *Pediatrics* 20:439, 1957.
17. Lyttle, J. D. Pneumococcic peritonitis in nephrosis. *Amer. J. Dis. Child.* 48:1171, 1934.
18. Pierce, A. K., Edmondson, E. B., McGee, G., Ketchersid, J., London, R. G., and Sanford, J. P. An analysis of factors predisposing to gram-negative bacillary necrotizing pneumonia. *Amer. Rev. Resp. Dis.* 94:309, 1966.
19. Goffinet, D. R., Glatstein, E. J., and Merigan, T. C. Herpes zoster-varicella infections and lymphoma. *Ann. Intern. Med.* 76:235, 1972.
20. Abramson, E., Wilson, D., and Arky, R. A. Rhinocerebral phycomycosis in association with diabetic ketoacidosis. *Ann. Intern. Med.* 66:735, 1967.
21. Levine, A. S., Graw, R. G., Jr., and Young, R. C. Management of infections in patients with leukemia and lymphoma: Current concepts and experimental approaches. *Seminars Hemat.* 9:141, 1972.
22. Bodey, G. P., Hart, J., and Frei, E. J., III. Studies of a patient isolator unit and prophylactic antibiotics in cancer: Chemotherapy. *Cancer* 22:1018, 1968.
23. Bodey, G. P. Fungal infections complicating acute leukemia. *J. Chronic. Dis.* 19:667, 1966.
24. Emmons, C. W., Binford, C. H., and Utz, J. P. *Medical Mycology* (2d ed.). Philadelphia: Lea & Febiger, 1970.
25. Littman, M. L., and Walter, J. E. Cryptococcosis: Current status. *Amer. J. Med.* 45:922, 1968.
26. Young, R. C., Bennett, J. E., Vogel, C. L., Carbone, P. P., and Devita, V. T. Aspergillosis: The spectrum of the disease in 98 patients. *Medicine* 49:147, 1970.
27. Armstrong, D., Young, L. S., Meyer, R. D., and Blevins, A. H. Infectious complications of neoplastic disease. *Med. Clin. N. Amer.* 55:729, 1971.
28. Muller, S. A., Hermann, E. C., Jr., and Winkelman, R. K. Herpes simplex infections in hematologic malignancies. *Amer. J. Med.* 52:102, 1972.
29. Weller, T. H. The cytomegaloviruses: Ubiquitous agents with protean clinical manifestations. *New Eng. J. Med.* 285:203, 267, 1971.

30. Krugman, S., and Ward, R. *Infectious Diseases of Children*. St. Louis: Mosby, 1968. Chap. 23, p. 314.
31. Theologides, A., and Kennedy, B. J. Toxoplasmic myocarditis and pericarditis (editorial). *Amer. J. Med.* 47:169, 1969.
32. Western, K. A., Perera, D. R., and Schultz, M. G. Pentamidine isethionate in the treatment of *Pneumocystis carinii* pneumonia. *Ann. Intern. Med.* 73:695, 1970.
33. Goodman, J. S., Kaufman, L., and Koenig, M. G. Diagnosis of cryptococcal meningitis: Value of immunologic detection of cryptococcal antigen. *New Eng. J. Med.* 285:432, 1971.
34. Hahn, H. D., and Beaty, H. N. Transtracheal aspiration in the evaluation of patients with pneumonia. *Ann. Intern. Med.* 72:183, 1970.
35. Goldstein, E., and Hoeprich, P. D. Problems in the diagnosis and treatment of systemic candidiasis. *J. Infect. Dis.* 125:190, 193, 1972.
36. Levin, S. The fungal skin test as a diagnostic hindrance. *J. Infect. Dis.* 122:343, 1970.
37. Han, T., and Sokol, J. E. Lymphocyte response to phytohemagglutinin in Hodgkin's disease. *Amer. J. Med.* 48:728, 1970.
38. Scott, T. F. M. Herpes Simplex. In T. B. Fitzpatrick, K. A. Arndt, W. H. Clark, A. Z. Eisen, E. J. Van Scott, and J. H. Vaughn (Eds.), *Dermatology in General Medicine*. New York: Blakiston Div., McGraw-Hill, 1971. Chap. 25, pp. 1878–1892.
39. Farber, S., and Wolbach, S. B. Intranuclear and cytoplasmic inclusions ("protozoan-like bodies") in the salivary glands and other organs of infants. *Amer. J. Path.* 8:123, 1932.
40. Schimpff, S., Saterlee, W., Young, V. M., and Serpick, A. Empiric therapy with carbenicillin and gentamicin for febrile patients with cancer and granulocytopenia. *New Eng. J. Med.* 284:1061, 1971.
41. Bodner, S. J., Koenig, M. G., and Goodman, J. S. Bacteremic *Bacteroides* infections. *Ann. Intern. Med.* 73:537, 1970.
42. Harvey, J. C., Cantrell, J. R., and Fisher, A. M. Actinomycosis: Its recognition and treatment. *Ann. Intern. Med.* 46:868, 1957.
43. Adams, A. R., Jackson, J. M., Scopa, J., Lane, G. K., and Wilson, R. Nocardiosis: Diagnosis and management with a report of three cases. *Med. J. Aust.* 1:669, 1971.
44. Andriole, V. T., and Kravetz, H. M. The use of amphotericin B in man. *J.A.M.A.* 180:269, 1962.
45. Fass, R. J., and Perkins, R. L. 5-Fluorocytosine in the treatment of cryptococcal and *Candida* mycoses. *Ann. Intern. Med.* 74:535, 1971.
46. Medoff, G., Comfort, M., and Kobayashi, G. S. Synergistic action of amphotericin B and 5-fluorocytosine against yeast-like organisms. *Proc. Soc. Exp. Biol. Med.* 138:571, 1971.
47. Hrynink, W., Foerster, J., Shojania, M., and Chow, A. Cytarabine for herpes virus infections. *J.A.M.A.* 219:715, 1972.
48. Center for Disease Control. Surveillance of requests for zoster immune globulin. *Morbid. Mortal. Weekly Rep.* 20:352, 1971.
49. Wingfield, W. L., Pollack, D., and Grunert, R. R. Therapeutic efficacy of Amantadine HCl and Rimantadine HCl in naturally occurring influenza A2 respiratory illness in man. *New Eng. J. Med.* 281:579, 1969.
50. Barbero, G., Gray, J., Scott, T. F. M., and Kempe, C. H. Vaccinia

gangrenosa treated with hyperimmune vaccinal gamma globulin. *Pediatrics* 16:609, 1955.

51. Bauer, D. J., Dumbell, K. R., Fox-Hulme, P., and Sadler, P. W. The chemotherapy of variola major infection. *Bull. W.H.O.* 26:727, 1962.
52. Kahoe, D. E., Jacobs, L., Berje, H. K., and McCullough, N. B. Acquired toxoplasmosis: Observations on two parasitologically proved cases treated with pyrimethamine and triple sulfonamides. *New Eng. J. Med.* 257:1274, 1957.
53. Kirby, H. B., Kenomore, B., and Guckian, J. C. *Pneumocystis carinii* pneumonia treated with pyrimethamine and sulfadiazine. *Ann. Intern. Med.* 75:505, 1971.
54. Robbins, J. B., Miller, R. H., Arean, V. M., and Pearson, H. A. Successful treatment of *Pneumocystis carinii* pneumonitis in a patient with congenital hypogammaglobulinemia. *New Eng. J. Med.* 272:708, 1965.
55. Grow, R. G., Henderson, E. S., and Perry, S. Leukocyte Procurement and Transfusion into Leukopenic Patients. In G. Mathe (Ed.), *White Blood Cell Transfusions.* Paris: Centre National de la Recherche Scientifique, 1970. P. 233.
56. Lawrence, H. S. Transfer factor and cellular immune deficiency disease. *New Eng. J. Med.* 283:411, 1970.
57. Good, R. A. Immunologic reconstitution: The achievement and its meaning. *Hospital Practice* 4:41, 1969.
58. Siegel, S., Henderson, E. S., Perry, S., and Levine, A. S. Protected environments in acute leukemia. *Blood* 38:803, 1971.

11 / STREPTOCOCCAL DISEASE

Leonard N. Newmark

THE IMPORTANCE of streptococcal infections and their sequelae cannot be overemphasized. The attack rates and social and economic impacts due to the morbidity of these infections justify their clinical prominence. There are some thirteen serologically distinct groups of streptococci classified on the basis of cell wall carbohydrates. Despite the fact that organisms of every strain may be responsible for local and systemic human diseases, group A streptococci cause most infections and are the sole cause of rheumatic fever and acute glomerulonephritis. This chapter outlines the diagnosis and treatment of streptococcal infections and emphasizes the importance of diagnosis and treatment in the prevention of rheumatic fever.

THE STREPTOCOCCUS

MORPHOLOGY AND COLONIES

Streptococci are members of the family Lactobacillaceae, genus *Streptococcus* [1]. They are spherical or ovoid; are rarely clumped, usually being arranged in long or short chains or in pairs, depending upon growth conditions; and are occasionally encapsulated. They are gram-positive, catalase negative, and insoluble in bile. (Bile solubility is characteristic of the pneumococcus.) The cells vary in size from 0.5 to 1.0 μ in diameter. They usually grow poorly on artificial media except those containing blood. Most species are facultatively anaerobic, but some are obligate anaerobes. Although most of the species are parasitic to man and animals, only a few are pathogenic. The organisms grow as small, rather delicate, grayish, opalescent colonies on blood agar plates. The colonies are circular but often have finely corrugated margins.

Classification

Three general forms of classification of streptococci are used, often leading to confusion among physicans.

1. Changes produced in blood-containing media: there are three types of reactions observed on blood agar plates. The alpha (α) type produces a greenish hue and only partial hemolysis of red cells surrounding the colony. This is characteristic of the viridans organisms. The beta (β) type produces a characteristic clear zone of hemolysis surrounding the colony. These are the hemolytic streptococci. The gamma (γ) organisms do not alter the red blood cells in the medium and are nonhemolytic.
2. Biologic characteristics form the basis of another type of classification. Aerobic streptococci are divided into four groups: pyogenic, viridans, enterococcus, and lactic groups. Members of each group share several common physiologic characteristics [1]. The relationships between Lancefield's serologic groups (see below) and several physiologic characteristics of streptococci are beautifully demonstrated in Table 64-1 of Gradwohl's manual [2].
3. The analysis of antigenic properties forms the basis of the third form of classification. The hemolytic streptococci can be serologically differentiated into completely separate groups utilizing the precipitin reaction [3]. This is possible because strains of each group elaborate a specific carbohydrate, the *C substance*. Groups of particular medical significance are: A, B, C, F, and G in the respiratory tract and D in the genitourinary tract. Although occasionally implicated, groups E, H, K, and O are not often responsible for disease. Further subdivisions of the group A streptococci have been achieved based on type-specific protein, the so-called M antigen. It is this protein that is responsible for virulence. Fortunately, a given streptococcal strain usually possesses a single M protein, and consequently the precipitin test yields a more specific reaction for identification. At least fifty-one separate M proteins have been identified.

The Hemolytic Streptococci

It is important to note that although the greatest number of human streptococcal infections are caused by group A organisms, which are nearly all β-hemolytic, groups B, C, F, G, and H also cause β-hemolysis. Furthermore, nonhemolytic group A streptococci also have been responsible for acute rheumatic fever. Therefore, the presence or absence of β-hemolysis on a blood agar plate is not always sufficient evidence of group A organisms or pathogenicity. Group A streptococci form two types of hemolysins: streptolysin O and S, the former being oxygen labile and the latter oxygen stable. Streptolysin O is antigenic, and the antistreptolysin O (ASO) serologic titer is useful in detecting recent group A infections. These organisms are all termed *Streptococcus pyogenes.* Fluorescent antibody studies are often used to delineate streptococcal groups.

Group B streptococci have definitely been causative in a number of serious infections. They have been isolated in empyema, septic arthritis, exudative pharyngitis, and in neonatal meningitis [4]. These organisms have been identified in 5% of apparently normal throats and frequently in the female external urogenitalia. Approximately 10% of pregnant women have been said to carry the organism in the genitalia, nipples, or throat. Organisms of this group may be suspected, in distinction to those of group A, because of the so-called double-zoned β-hemolysis and the larger diameter of the colonies on blood agar plates. Group B organisms have been termed *Strep. agalactiae.*

Group C streptococci (*Strep. equisimilis*) also cause β-hemolysis but are rarely implicated in human infections. Group F streptococci are slowly growing β-hemolytic organisms which form very small, transparent colonies. They have been isolated from routine pharyngeal cultures and are thought to be responsible for a small number of upper respiratory tract infections. Group G organisms rarely account for tonsillitis, subacute endocarditis, or urinary tract infections. Group H organisms were originally isolated from vegetations in a patient with subacute endocarditis, but they are most unusual pathogens [5].

The Viridans Streptococci

The characteristic green discoloration surrounding colonies of α-hemolytic streptococci is the hallmark of the so-called *Strep.* viridans. These organisms are members of the normal flora of human throats and are occasionally isolated from the colon. They are the most frequent cause of subacute bacterial endocarditis [6]. In the past, *Diplococcus pneumoniae* was included in the viridans group, but because *D. pneumoniae* is bile soluble, it is usually considered separately.

The Enterococci

A common polysaccharide antigen is shared by these group D organisms. Although all forms of hemolysis are found, generally they do not produce hemolysins. Members of this group which are commonly isolated are *Strep. faecalis, Strep. faecalis* variant *liquefaciens,* and *Strep. faecalis* variant *zymogenes.* These organisms are usually isolated from the intestinal lumen, the genitourinary tract, and the saliva. Despite their omnipresence in health, they are causative in some urinary tract infections and commonly in subacute bacterial endocarditis. Since these organisms have been frequently insensitive to penicillin, in distinction to group A organisms, identification is mandatory for appropriate therapy. Indeed, effective therapy may require penicillin in addition to another antibiotic.

The Anaerobic Streptococci

These common inhabitants of normal orifices are frequently responsible for puerperal sepsis, necrosis of injured muscle, gangrene of the lungs, hepatic abscesses, otitis media and mastoiditis, and urinary tract infections. They play a major role in the pathogenesis of septic abortions. They are commonly found in the mouth, vagina, and large intestine. Smaller than most other streptococci, these organisms are usually obligate anaerobes but sometimes are microaerophilic. They produce a characteristic foul or putrid odor in exudates. They are usually not easily recovered, and their presence in any body fluid is prima facie evidence of infection.

THE ISOLATION AND IDENTIFICATION OF STREPTOCOCCI

In office practice, most specimens are obtained from the oropharynx or nasopharynx, vagina, coughed sputa, exudates from skin lesions, or pus. In the hospital environment, blood, cerebrospinal fluid, both transudates and exudates from lesions in viscera, and surgical tissue specimens may be added to this list. Three general methods of identifying streptococci are available to the clinician.

1. A microscopical search may be made for gram-positive cocci arranged in both short and long chains. This is obviously hardly opti-

mal and often may actually confuse even the most astute clinician with training in microbiology.

2. Commercial laboratories or neighboring hospital facilities are not only available but are recommended for use by those who do not wish to establish their own culture facilities. Specimens of nasopharyngeal or oropharyngeal swabs may be placed in a nonnutrient, semisolid, commercially available transport media. The Stuart medium is ideal for this purpose [7] and is available from most major biologic supply houses. It is important to be certain that the swabs used have been commercially prepared for this purpose in order to eliminate preservatives, or that one of several cotton and wood "decontaminating" procedures is employed if the standard wooden applicator with a cotton tip is used. Commercial and hospital laboratories use a variety of isolation and identification techniques far too complex for office use. Fluorescent antibody (FA) techniques for identification of group A streptococci are very popular in large city and state laboratories.

3. Streptococci may be readily cultured in a private office and sufficiently identified with an investment in 5% sheep blood agar plates, an alcohol or gas lamp, a platinum inoculating wire loop, an inexpensive tabletop incubator, and bacitracin discs. Several models of incubators are available for less than $100.

Group A streptococci are more sensitive to bacitracin than other β-hemolytic streptococci. This characteristic may be readily applied to the use of blood agar plates for identification.

Screening identification may be readily accomplished in the following manner: the posterior oropharynx, tonsils, or any other possible source of infection is swabbed. The swab is immediately passed gently over one-sixth to one-quarter of the surface of a blood agar plate. (In the author's office, duplicate swabs are immersed in transport media and sent to the municipal health department, where FA screening is performed at no charge.) The plate is then completely streaked with a sterile loop and the agar is stabbed at least a dozen times to facilitate the growth of subsurface hemolytic colonies. A single bacitracin disc is centrally placed on the agar, and the plate is then incubated at 37°C. for approximately 24 hours. It requires little acumen to discern hemolytic colonies. Growth of subcultured group A colonies is inhibited by the bacitracin discs in a zone of 12 to 17 mm. The disc test is reliable 90 to 95% of the time in streptococcal disease but less so in carrier states [8].

Only early in streptococcal pharyngitis or tonsillitis will organisms be found in quantity. Nonetheless, recovery of at least ten colonies will be the rule, and over fifty colonies at least half the time. If fewer than ten colonies are grown, the patient may well be a carrier who has developed pharyngitis from another infecting agent, usually a virus [9]. Carriers of hemolytic colonies that are not group A usually grow fewer than ten colonies. If more than ten colonies of β-hemolytic group A streptococci are demonstrated on blood agar plates, the patient should be considered infected and treated appropriately.

THE ORGANISM, THE HOST, AND CLINICAL SYNDROMES

It would be intellectually satisfying, if not ideal, if one could now describe the relationship of streptococcal cellular components, proteins with antigenic properties, and enzymes and toxins produced by the streptococci to disease patterns. Certainly the literature is replete with accurate and reliable data on the nature not only of the organism and its products and components in vitro but also in vivo. There remains, however, no common denominator for describing the pathogenesis of streptococci and the infections they may cause. The organism and the human host interaction are astonishingly complex. To illustrate, an epidemic of scarlet fever proved to be caused by a specific streptococcal type occurred on one military post while, despite the presence of the same organism, another post had no cases at all. Diseases caused by streptococci are, in lieu of precise pathogenicity, classified by the primary anatomic site involved by infection, if suppurative, and by historical description if the disease is the result of streptococcal toxins or antigen-antibody reactions.

The M protein elaborated by group A organisms is apparently of particular significance, and the immunity resulting from infection is type-specific for that M protein. These antibodies are now known to remain in the human host for years following infection, and reinfection by the same M serotype is most unusual. Interestingly, the quantity of M protein elaborated correlates well with the organism's ability to resist phagocytosis. Acquired immunity to many strains may account for the age incidence in the epidemiology of pharyngitis produced by group A organisms.

In addition to type-specific M protein, hyaluronidase, streptolysin O, streptokinase (fibrinolysin), and proteinases including enzyme hydrolyzing diphosphopyridine nucleotide (DPNase) and deoxyribonuclease (DNase), all of which are antigenic, are produced by group A streptococci. These products probably contribute to the characteristics pathologically manifested by the organism. Streptokinase has been implicated in causing thin pus and, with hyaluronidase, may be responsible for the rapid dissemination of the organism through the host's tissues, as happens in cellulitis or erysipelas.

THE EPIDEMIOLOGY OF STREPTOCOCCAL INFECTIONS

From a purely numerical point of view, pharyngitis, tonsillitis, and scarlet fever dominate group A infections. The bulk of these infections occur in the pediatric groups of 5 to 15 years of age, but certainly both younger and older people are susceptible. Of epidemiologic importance is the fact that man is the only established source of these microorganisms for respiratory infections [9]. Although outbreaks of streptococcal infections have been reported as a result of contaminated food or milk, there are no known important reservoirs other than humans [10]. Organisms found on dirt, dust, and clothing are not usually infective and apparently produce no disease when inoculated into the throats of human volunteers [11]. Approximately 50% of the members of any given household may be expected to become infected from the introduction of an untreated child into the household. Unlike many other microorganisms, streptococci are transmitted by direct or intimate contact with another person with pharyngitis or tonsillitis, and not by airborne droplets. Unfortunately, many infections are totally ignored because of the lack of subjective complaints, but these children and adults become the carriers responsible for spreading the infection since infectivity bears little relationship to symptomatology.

In a susceptible host, a few organisms not removed by the mucosa of the upper respiratory tract form a small locus of infection which may quickly involve nasopharyngeal and oropharyngeal lymphoid tissue. In approximately 60% of people, symptoms develop at this time, but another 20% may remain without subjective complaints. In the first 24 to 48 hours following inoculation, large numbers of organisms can be cultured from both the nasopharynx and the nares. Despite the absence of treatment, both the symptoms and recoverability of the organism rapidly recede. In three to four weeks, swab cultures will usually yield fewer than ten colonies from the oropharynx and nasopharynx. At this level the organisms may persist for weeks or months in a carrier state. Type-specific immunity develops within three to eight weeks after infection and persists for an indefinite period. It is interesting to note that although antibiotic therapy inhibits the production of type-specific antibodies, it has not been shown to be of clinically practical importance.

Geographic factors and season may also influence population

densities and thus the rate of infection. In military posts and high-density civilian populations, particularly in poverty areas, infection rates are highest.

In the United States the peak incidence of streptococcal pharyngeal infections is between December and May and of pyoderma in the summer. This coincides with the peak incidences of acute rheumatic fever (ARF) and glomerulonephritis, respectively.

Unlike all other sequelae of streptococcal infections, scarlet fever stands alone. Strains causing this rash are peculiarly susceptible to a lysogenic bacteriophage which produces an erythrogenic toxin. Consequently, although epidemics of streptococcal pharyngitis are frequent, the scarlet fever is sporadic.

Streptococcal glomerulonephritis and ARF have occupied the interest of many observers. It now appears almost incontrovertible that there are both nephritogenic and nonnephritogenic strains of group A streptococci. In contrast, there appears to be no nonrheumatogenic strain; even nonhemolytic group A infection has been implicated in ARF. In closed populations, epidemics of exudative pharyngitis due to group A organisms are followed by an approximate attack rate of 3% of ARF. This was demonstrated to be irrespective of M-protein serotype [12]. Since Rammelkamp's work, variations in attack rates of acute rheumatic fever in civilian populations have been found to be influenced more by virulence of the strain and numerical occurrence than the qualitative differences in the infecting strains [13]. Indeed, it was suggested that there may be a quantitative threshold of streptococcal pharyngitis beyond which ARF does not occur. It appears well founded now that suppurative complications are more prone to occur in people who still have tonsils and adenoids, and recurrences of rheumatic fever are far more common in these people. In fact, the size of tonsillar tissue has been correlated with recurrence rates [14].

To support the concept that there are antigenic differences between rheumatogenic and nephritogenic strains, it has been observed that ARF is almost exclusively a complication of pharyngeal infection. Acute rheumatic fever has not, on the other hand, been shown to be the result of streptococcal pyoderma. Pyoderma streptococci colonize the pharynx also, and glomerulonephritis may occur after either throat or skin infections with nephritogenic strains. Most rheumatogenic strains do not parasitize the skin. Strains of M serotypes 1, 3, 5, 6, 18, 19, and 24 have thus far not been shown to cause acute glomerulonephritis. Types 12, 14, 49, 52, 53, 54, 55, 56, 57, 58, 59, 60, and 61 have been demonstrated in epidemic streptococcal glomerulonephritis. Clinical aspects of scarlet fever, ARF, and streptococcal glomerulonephritis have not substantially changed in the past few years and are thoroughly covered in many medical texts and reviews.

TREATMENT AND PROPHYLAXIS

There are several important reasons for treating all infections. Among the most applicable to streptococcal infections are (1) to abbreviate the acute phase of the illness, (2) to prevent sequelae of the infection, and (3) to reduce or substantially prevent dissemination of the infecting microorganisms to other susceptible individuals. Seldom mentioned in considering streptococcal illnesses, particularly pharyngitis and tonsillitis, is the fact that only if antibiotics are begun within the first 24 hours does the treatment in any way shorten or minimize symptomatology. Since this is almost always impossible in clinical practice, there is no reason to initiate therapy with a potentially hazardous drug until a bacteriologic diagnosis can be secured with a significant degree of confidence.

Appropriate antibiotic therapy virtually eliminates otitis media, mastoiditis, sinusitis, cervical adenitis, and peritonsillar cellulitis, so the previously observed mortality with these complications has been strikingly reduced. Voluminous data are now available to demonstrate that appropriate therapy of streptococcal infections will prevent ARF, and thus presumably rheumatic valvular disease, in nearly 100% of patients if treatment is initiated early and in 90% of patients if it is instituted within nine days of onset. In various studies 10, 33, 58, 92, and 100% of rheumatic fever patients have demonstrated latent periods of less than one, two, three, four, and five weeks, respectively [9].

Unfortunately, the saga is considerably different for streptococcal acute glomerulonephritis. Despite the conclusions of Rammelkamp and his co-workers, subsequent statistical analyses have failed to prove that penicillin therapy altered the incidence of acute glomerulonephritis. The current available data suggest that penicillin may slightly reduce the risk of nephritis in patients recovering from pyoderma but not in patients recovering from pharyngitis. There are unfortunately an insufficient number of statistically significant reports available at this writing. Weinstein and Frock pointed out that because of the outstanding efficacy of penicillin and other new antibiotics in curing streptococcal infections and virtually eradicating suppurative complications, the withholding of adequate antibiotic therapy to obtain statistically valid data is difficult if not totally impossible to justify [15]. It should be apparent nonetheless that despite insufficient data regarding glomerulonephritis prophylaxis, all streptococcal infections will still require adequate therapy for two reasons: (1) infectious complications are almost eliminated and morbidity strikingly reduced, and (2) the pool of dissemination of these microorganisms, even nephritogenic strains, is substantially diminished.

Several guidelines accrue from these data. All patients with streptococcal infections should be adequately treated, that is, the microorganism should be eliminated. Any febrile respiratory infection with attendant painful deglutition, tender cervical lymphadenopathy, and pharyngeal exudate should be suspect. Whenever possible, appropriate cultures should be obtained. In addition, a total leukocyte count may be very helpful. If counts are less than 10,000, the culture results may be awaited, but if greater than 10,000, therapy should be started. If cultures cannot be reasonably obtained, therapy should be instituted. When one member of a household has been shown to have streptococcal infection, therapy should be extended to any other member who manifests symptoms. Contacts whose symptoms developed prior to the patient's should also be treated despite their apparent recovery. Adequate data have shown that clinical recovery from streptococcal pharyngitis is a useless criterion for adequate treatment. Only after the organisms are no longer culturable are the attack rates of rheumatic fever altered.

Further data will establish whether the new antibiotics are acceptable forms of therapy, but for the present, penicillin remains the drug of choice in all streptococcal infections (except enterococcal streptococci). It appears that a single injection of benzathine penicillin remains optimal, 1.2 million units for adults and 0.6 to 0.9 million units for children, to eliminate 95 to 99% of streptococcal infections. If parenteral penicillin is not chosen, oral penicillin may be used. Penicillin G or phenoxymethyl penicillin (V) should be used in doses of 250,000 and 200,000 units, respectively, three to four times daily for ten days. Erythromycin, 250 mg. every 6 hours for ten days, will be effective in up to 90% of cases when penicillin cannot be used. A full ten days of therapy must be emphasized to the patient. Tetracyclines are less effective due to resistant strains, and sulfa does not eliminate the carrier state so should not be used.

In patients with previous acute rheumatic fever, monthly parenteral penicillin (benzathine), 1.2 million units, or daily oral penicillin, 200,000 units, should be used indefinitely.

REFERENCES

1. Breed, R. S., Murray, E. G. D., and Smith, N. R. (Eds.). *Bergey's Manual of Determinative Bacteriology* (7th ed.). Baltimore: Williams & Wilkins, 1957.
2. Frankel, S., Reitman, S., and Sonnenwirth, A. C. (Eds.). *Gradwohl's Clinical Laboratory Methods and Diagnosis* (7th ed.). St. Louis: Mosby, 1970.
3. Lancefield, R. C. Preparation and properties of protein (R antigen)

occurring in streptococci of group A, type 28 and in certain streptococci of other serological groups. *J. Exp. Med.* 96:83, 1952.
4. Harper, I. A. The importance of group B streptococci as human pathogens in the British Isles. *J. Clin. Path.* 24:438, 1971.
5. Hare, R. Classification of haemolytic streptococci from nose and throat of normal human beings by means of precipitin and biochemical tests. *J. Path. Bact.* 41:499, 1935.
6. Robinovich, S., Smith, I. M., and January, L. E. The changing pattern of bacterial endocarditis. *Med. Clin. N. Amer.* 52:1091, 1968.
7. Stuart, R. D. Transport medium for specimens in public health bacteriology. *Public Health Rep.* 74:431, 1959.
8. Jelinkova, J., and Rotta, J. The bacitracin test for recognition of group A streptococci. *Int. J. System. Bact.* 17:297, 1967.
9. Rammelkamp, C. H., Jr., and Morson, T. P. Streptococcal infections: Why it's important to diagnose and treat them quickly. *Med. Times* 99:48, 1971.
10. Rammelkamp, C. H., Jr. *Harvey Lectures,* Epidemiology of streptococcal infections. Series 51, 1955–56. New York: Academic, 1957. Pp. 113–142.
11. Stollerman, G. H. Group A Streptococcal Infections. In P. B. Beeson and W. McDermott (Eds.), *Textbook of Medicine* (12th ed.). Philadelphia: Saunders, 1967. Pp. 511–521.
12. Rammelkamp, C. H., Jr., Denny, F. W., and Wannamaker, L. W. Studies on the Epidemiology of Rheumatic Fever in the Armed Services. In L. Thomas (Ed.), *Rheumatic Fever.* Minneapolis: University of Minnesota Press, 1952.
13. Stollerman, G. H. Rheumatogenic and nephritogenic streptococci. *Circulation* 43:915, 1971.
14. Feinstein, A. R., and Levitt, M. The role of tonsils in predisposing to streptococcal infections and recurrences of rheumatic fever. *New Eng. J. Med.* 282:814, 1970.
15. Weinstein, L., and LeFrock, J. Does antimicrobial therapy of streptococcal pharyngitis or pyoderma alter the risk of glomerulonephritis? *J. Infect. Dis.* 124:229, 1971.

12 / VENEREAL DISEASE

J. Joseph Marr

In spite of efficacious therapy and a reasonably good understanding of the pathogenesis and epidemiology, venereal diseases have increased in incidence. This increase has occurred in all age groups, but it has been especially marked in the younger segment of our society. The reasons for this increase are generally conceded to be an alteration in moral outlook among the population in general as well as an increase in travel; whether these reasons are correct is open to question. In this country lack of public education probably plays a significant role, especially in our higher population density urban areas. A benign neglect on the part of the medical profession has also contributed to the prevalence of these diseases.

SYPHILIS

Syphilis is a chronic infectious multisystem disease caused by *Treponema pallidum;* its transmission is almost always through venereal contact, with rapid systemic spread. The disease remains widespread despite excellent methods for its diagnosis and treatment. During the 1950's and early 1960's, there was a marked upsurge in infectious primary and secondary syphilis in this country, reaching a peak in 1965, when over 25,000 cases were reported [1]. The number of reported cases underwent a decline until 1970 and then began to rise again [2]. The true incidence of syphilis is doubtless much higher than that which is reported; for example, a questionnaire sent to over 200,000 practicing physicians in the United States asked if they had treated and reported any venereal disease during a three-month period in 1968. Two-thirds of the physicians responded, and the results indicated that although private physicians treat over 80% of all cases of infectious syphilis, only 12% of these cases are reported to public health authorities. The authors of this questionnaire, using this data, were able to calculate a true annual incidence of infectious syphilis for 1968 of 75,000 cases, or four times the reported number [3]. Syphilis remains the third most commonly reported infectious disease in the United States, and in 1970 there were an estimated 200,000 new cases.

This disease is most prevalent in young adults in large urban centers, with 62% of cases occurring in persons between the ages 15 and 25. Propagation is facilitated by the properties of the agent, its mode of transmission, and by social and environmental factors. The pattern of promiscuity and of heterosexual and homosexual relations has altered so that in some urban areas about 25 to 50% of all males with syphilis have acquired it through a homosexual contact. Each person with infectious syphilis has had an average of 4.6 recent contacts, 2 of whom were infected.

Following the implantation and local multiplication of *T. pallidum* and extension of the infection to the lymph nodes, treponemas spread rapidly to all tissues. Human syphilis therefore rapidly becomes a systemic disease. Although the agent itself does not multiply in the bloodstream, numerous metastatic foci are set up within the body and in the skin, mucosae, and nervous system. Multiplication continues there for several weeks. During this time the patient has no visible lesion or systemic symptoms; his blood is, however, infectious. From two to six weeks after the initial implantation, the primary lesion appears. This sore may be single or multiple and is usually not painful unless secondary infection has occurred. The lesions of secondary syphilis appear about two or three weeks after the onset of the primary lesion, and in perhaps a third of the patients the lesions of primary and secondary syphilis coexist, involving all portions of the integument. Most organisms in the integument and internal organs are killed, but sometimes they become only temporarily inactivated (latent) and give rise to further manifestations.

In the untreated disease further secondary episodes occur in about 25% of the patients within the first four years and generally within two years. With increasing duration of infection the hematogenous "showers" of treponemas become less frequent and involve decreasing numbers of organisms. The cutaneous lesions tend to group and localize, and a lesion may occur solitarily until the mucocutaneous system no longer responds with visible pathologic changes. The further course of untreated infection is documented in the data from the University Clinic in Oslo, where about 1,100 patients diagnosed as having early syphilis remained untreated under hospital conditions and underwent extensive follow-up evaluations. In the last investigation, fifty years after the original infection had occurred, late, so-called benign syphilis had occurred in 15%, cardiovascular syphilis in 10%, and neurosyphilis in 6.5% of these patients [4]. Ten percent had died as a direct consequence of their disease, and in about two-thirds latency continued indefinitely after subsidence of the secondary attacks. The remainder of the lives of these individuals was unattended by any major physical or mental consequence of the disease.

These features of the host-parasite relationship in syphilis raise questions regarding the mechanisms involved in the pathogenesis of the lesions and their nature in both early and late disease and illustrate the remarkable response of the host to the invading pathogen. The reasons for the persistence of these organisms despite an apparently adequate immunologic response remains one of the major unanswered questions of infectious disease research today.

IMMUNOLOGY

The modification of the natural course of syphilis heralds the immune response of the host. The waning treponemiasis, the decrease in demonstrable treponemas in late lesions, and the presence of presumed resistance to superinfection all indicate that the immune response is significant in bringing about cure or suppression of the disease. Knowledge regarding the effector mechanisms in the host responses and the role of humoral and cell-mediated immunity in the natural history of this disease is meager. Despite this, the serologic diagnosis of syphilis has become increasingly sophisticated and represents a major clinical and public health tool for recognition and control of the disease. The various serologic tests devolve directly from the antibody response mustered by the host. These antibodies, although multiple, are of two main types.

1. Nonspecific antibodies (reagins) are directed against lipid antigens of the treponemas or against a lipid antigen that results from the interaction of host and parasite and develop about five weeks after infection. Tests for reagins are nontreponemal tests and are often described as serologic tests for syphilis. The cardiolipin-lecithin antigens used in the nontreponemal tests are found in many normal tissues and sometimes give a positive test even though the patient does

not have syphilis. The reaginic antibody declines as the disease moves toward latency and may fall below detectable levels in late disease. It is affected by therapy in the early phase of syphilis, so that a rising titer is a useful gauge of disease activity although of limited value as an indicator of immunity. There is no evidence that reagin has a protective role in the host. Its pathogenic significance is unknown, and it is presumed to be an antibody formed in response to small amounts of cardiolipin lost from host cells in the pathologic process [5].

2. Specific antitreponemal antibodies, which are measured by a variety of treponemal tests. These use one of a variety of preparations of the treponema itself as the antigen, and a positive test is usually quite specific for past or present infection. Of the treponemal antibodies, the immobilizing antibody appears to be the most important, although agglutinating treponemal antibodies also appear. These specific antibodies appear two to three months after infection but can persist for life as an indicator of past infection. The development of these antibodies generally reflects the acquisition of true host resistance, although the evidence is somewhat equivocal that they have a protective role.

As in most infections, the principal antibodies in syphilis belong to immunoglobulins of the IgM or IgG classes. Antibody demonstrated by reagin tests may belong to either class; IgM is produced early in the infection, and IgG appears later. The immobilizing antibody is always IgG. The IgG antibodies can pass the placenta, in contrast to IgM, so the presence of IgM in the serum of a newborn suggests local formation of antibodies and active prenatal infection. The presence of IgG antibodies in postnatal serum is indicative of infection in the mother. The IgG antibody also passes the blood–brain barrier when the meninges are inflamed, and this is the reason why serodiagnostic tests that mainly identify IgG antibody are preferred in examining the cerebrospinal fluid.

Cell-mediated immunity manifests itself as a delayed hypersensitivity, demonstrable by the response to intradermally injected antigen after 12 to 48 hours. Although knowledge is limited at this time, cell-mediated immunity does not appear to play a major role during the secondary eruptions of syphilis [6]. It is believed to be important in the formation of gummatous lesions.

Immunopathologic mechanisms causing tissue damage in syphilis are poorly understood. Multiple humoral antibodies circulate in all phases of the disease, antigen is present, and antigen-antibody complexes may have some pathogenic significance, although a direct cytotoxic effect on host cells has not been demonstrated. These mechanisms have been suggested by some of the manifestations engendered by syphilis, particularly paroxysmal cold hemoglobinuria and membranous glomerulonephritis (syphilitic nephrosis). At present the clinical and laboratory findings only illustrate the capacity of immunocompetent cell systems to react to antigenic stimuli in the early phase of syphilis and to generate protection against further metastatic spread and superinfection with the same pathogen. The human host can contain the infection during latency by establishing an equilibrium between the treponemas and the immune forces, as evidenced by the relatively infrequent disturbance of this equilibrium manifesting itself as late symptomatic disease.

Serologic Tests for Syphilis

The nontreponemal tests are the most widely used and are of two general types: flocculation and complement fixation. The Venereal Disease Research Laboratory slide test (VDRL) is the most commonly used flocculation test and the Kolmer the common complement-fixation test employed today. These are easily performed and quantitated, are inexpensive, and remain the standard tests for screening purposes. They also are used in following the serologic response to treatment, since the titer declines when the disease is eradicated much more rapidly than does the fluorescent treponemal antibody absorption titer (see third paragraph following) [6, 7].

A difficulty with these reagin tests is that they are not always specific for syphilis. False-positive reactions are not uncommon; their incidence varies from 20% in the study of Fiumara [8] to about 5% in the series presented by Moore and Mohr [9], and they usually have a titer of 1:1 to 1:4. Most acute false-positive reactions occur after a variety of infections or immunizations and are generally of little importance. Approximately one-fourth of the chronic reactors have serious underlying disease, usually systemic lupus erythematosus or a related connective tissue disease. Common clinical situations which have been confirmed as causes of acute false-positive reactions are smallpox vaccinations, atypical pneumonia, and narcotic addiction (this may approximate 20 to 25% [10]). Aging is another common cause of chronic false-positive VDRL tests; for example, 1.7% of 10,000 men of ages 55 to 60 and 9 to 10% of patients who were 70 to 89 years of age showed a positive VDRL [11, 12]. These reactions in older persons are generally of a very low titer and associated with increased total globulins, antinuclear antibodies, and rheumatoid factor.

Because of the aforementioned difficulties, a number of methods have been devised to test for antibodies which are specific for syphilis. The first treponemal test, the *T. pallidum* immobilization test (TPI), measures the ability of antibody and complement to immobilize a suspension of living treponemas. This test is expensive and is performed in only a few laboratories. The presence of antibiotics in a serum specimen will invalidate it, since the antibiotic will also inactivate motile treponemas. Reactivity to the TPI test develops slowly: two-thirds of patients with primary and one-third of those with secondary syphilis have a negative test [13]. Another test is the Reiter protein complement-fixation test (RPCF). This is cheaper and more easily performed than the TPI, but it has fallen out of use because it is reactive in no more than half of persons with late syphilis.

The most important treponemal test has resulted from the application of immunofluorescent techniques. The fluorescent treponemal antibody (FTA) test employs a strain of *T. pallidum* as the antigen; this is placed on a glass slide and a sample of the patient's serum is added. Antibody which then attaches to the treponemas is detected by the addition of fluorescein-labeled antihuman gamma globulin and visualization by fluorescent microscopy. This test has undergone a number of modifications and is now carried out using absorbed serum and is known as the fluorescent treponemal antibody absorption test (FTA-ABS). A 1:5 dilution of the patient's serum is absorbed with an extract of a culture of the nonpathogenic Reiter strain of treponemas in order to remove group antibody directed against antigens which are common to *T. pallidum*, the Reiter strain, and other nonpathogenic oral and genital treponemas that are normal saprophytes in man [14]. The present FTA-ABS test appears to have the best features of all the versions, being reactive even in the primary stage in most cases of syphilis, and so far having been falsely positive only on rare occasions. In these latter instances, the reaction is not truly falsely positive since the staining pattern is different from that seen with a normally reactive serum. The FTA-ABS test for syphilis has replaced the TPI and is a standard treponemal test in most state health laboratories.

The comparative values of the available tests for syphilis are listed in Table 12-1. The superiority of the FTA-ABS technique is evident. It becomes reactive first in early syphilis and remains reactive for many years in old or treated syphilis. A reactive FTA-ABS test is thus a good indication that the patient has had syphilis, but it does not indicate clinical activity or necessity for treatment. Although the VDRL titer rises somewhat more slowly in early disease, its more rapid fall after treatment makes it the best test for following the response to treatment [7]. It is important to note that since the VDRL test is non-

TABLE 12-1 / Reactivity of Serologic Tests for Syphilis at Various Clinical Stages

Classification of Disease	Number of Tests	Percent Reactive		
		FTA-ABS	TPI	VDRL
Primary	191	85	56	78
Secondary	270	99	94	97
Late	117	95	92	77
Latent	954	95	94	74
Normal—no disease	384	1	0	0

FTA-ABS = fluorescent treponemal antibody absorption test; TPI = *Treponema pallidum* immobilization test; VDRL = Venereal Disease Research Laboratory slide test.
SOURCE: adapted from Deacon et al. [35] and Sparling [36].

reactive in as many as a third of the cases of late syphilis, it is clearly necessary to perform the more sensitive FTA-ABS test in any patient in whom there is a clinical suspicion of late syphilis of the central nervous or cardiovascular systems.

Serology in Congenital Syphilis. The diagnosis of congenital syphilis is not difficult when the infant has the typical clinical signs of rhinitis, rash, anemia, hepatosplenomegaly, jaundice, or osteochondritis, especially if dark-field positive lesions are present. Diagnosis becomes much more difficult when an apparently normal neonate is serologically positive; this may be due either to passive transfer of maternal antibody or to active infection. When confronted with this problem the physician may do a VDRL antibody titer on the infant using the infant's serum; the titer of passively transferred antibody in the infant serum is usually not greater than the titer in the mother's serum, and it generally declines rather rapidly during the first three months of life. The situation may be complicated, however, by the fact that the mother who acquires syphilis late in pregnancy may give birth to an infant with a negative serologic test for syphilis yet one who develops clinically manifest syphilis at about one to two months of age. In the former situation the physician must either delay treatment until he has observed serial decreases in the antibody titer or administer therapy to a number of nonsyphilitic infants. In the latter situation the physician may not treat a number of infants with negative VDRL tests yet who in fact are incubating syphilis.

Because of these quandaries there has been much interest generated by the development of a more sensitive and specific test for congenital syphilis. It is now known that the earliest antibody response of an individual is found in the IgM fraction of the immune globulins and only later do IgG globulins begin to increase. Under normal conditions only IgG is transferred across the placenta, so that the presence of elevated amounts of IgM in umbilical cord or fetal blood is well correlated with active fetal infection [15]. Total serum IgM is often elevated in congenital syphilis and may actually precede the onset of clinical disease [16]. The FTA-ABS test has been modified to use fluorescein-labeled antihuman IgM to detect specific anti-treponemal IgM antibodies. The sensitivity of this IgM FTA-ABS test in congenital syphilis has been well documented [17].

Treatment of Syphilis

The following are the current recommendations of the U.S. Public Health Service for the treatment of syphilis [18].

1. Primary and secondary syphilis and case contacts: 2.4 million units of benzathine penicillin in two injections at a single visit.
2. Latent syphilis (early and late): if no spinal fluid examination is performed, then the patient should be treated as though he has tertiary syphilis (see below). If the spinal fluid is not reactive, than 2.4 million units of benzathine penicillin at a single visit is sufficient therapy.
3. Tertiary syphilis and latent syphilis with a positive spinal fluid serology: 2.4 million units of benzathine penicillin initially, then 2.4 million units each week for the next three weeks. The total dose is 9.6 million units over a twenty-eight-day period.
4. Syphilis in pregnancy: treated as above, depending upon the stage, and during subsequent pregnancies patients are always retreated if there is any doubt regarding the adequacy of previous therapy. The newborn child is, of course, followed clinically and serologically for evidence of congenital syphilis.
5. Patients allergic to penicillin should be given tetracycline in a total dose of 30 gm. administered over ten to fifteen days. This is approximately as effective as penicillin. In the treatment of late syphilis tetracycline has not been as extensively evaluated, but it is recommended that a total dose of 60–80 gm. be administered [19]. Although the potential dangers from the use of tetracycline during pregnancy are small, erythromycin is the preferred drug in treating the pregnant patient with syphilis. It should be given as 500 mg. every 6 hours for a full twenty days.

Persisting Treponemas in Seronegative Syphilis. Physicians have long been comforted by the knowledge that penicillin, when properly administered, is an efficacious therapy for syphilis. Information has now begun to appear in the literature which may challenge this belief and raise new questions about the host-parasite relationship in late syphilis. The first apparent documentation of persistence of pathogenic *T. pallidum* in man after adequate penicillin therapy was by Collart et al. [20]. They removed lymph nodes from five patients with late syphilis and transferred them to normal rabbits. In two of the recipient rabbits dark-field positive testicular lesions developed. Smith's group in Miami, Florida, has demonstrated spiral organisms in the aqueous humor, cerebrospinal fluid, brain, and other tissues of several patients who had clinical evidence for nervous system or ocular syphilis, many of whom had negative serologic tests [21, 22]. In most cases the organisms were seen by dark-field or immunofluorescent microscopy; in only a few was infection successfully transferred to animals. The most impressive report was of three patients who had clinical evidence of syphilis of the eye, or tertiary syphilis involving the aorta, spinal cord, or liver, but all of whom had negative or equivocal serologic tests for syphilis [22]. Animals inoculated with cerebrospinal fluid and extracts of these tissues developed dark-field positive lesions. It should be emphasized that only those reports which contain successful animal infectivity experiments should be given serious consideration, since it has recently been demonstrated by this same group that falsely positive immunofluorescent stains can be produced at etch marks and water marks on the glass slides used for serologic tests [23].

The picture that emerges is not entirely clear, but it does seem reasonable to conclude that there has been a small number of isolations of *T. pallidum* documented by positive animal transfer from treated patients, particularly those with late neurosyphilis or ocular syphilis. Some of these patients had no serologic evidence for syphilis, including a negative FTA-ABS test. Whether or not these individuals have some defect in their immune system, particularly the cellular immune system, is not known. These studies do emphasize the fact that late syphilis can occur even if all serologic tests are negative. It does not seem indicated, however, to recommend a general change in the amount of penicillin used to treat late syphilis, since even very large amounts have not eradicated treponemas from many individuals. This is particularly true in symptomatic neurosyphilis, where progression of the disease is relatively common despite antibiotic therapy. When one considers the low serum levels of penicillin achieved with benzathine penicillin and the poor penetration of penicillin into the uninflamed eye and cerebrospinal fluid, it should not be too surprising that spirochetes can be isolated from the eyes and spinal fluid of a small number of treated patients with late syphilis. These cases may simply reflect too little of the drug given too late in the disease and not necessarily the development of penicillin-resistant mutants of *T. pallidum*. The best answer to the problem of the treatment of late syphilis remains, therefore, the proper treatment of the disease in its earliest stages.

GONORRHEA

Gonorrhea is an infection of the mucous membrane of the urethra and genital tract caused by *Neisseria gonorrhoeae*. Infection is almost always the result of sexual contact, and following invasion of the genitourinary tract organisms may spread to extragenital sites to cause arthritis, endocarditis, and meningitis. Gonorrhea is the most commonly reported communicable disease in this country, with an estimated 2 million new cases occurring in 1970. The number of new cases appears to be increasing at a rate of 10 to 15% per year. There are several factors inherent in the nature of gonorrhea which prevent control: its short incubation period, the absence of natural or acquired resistance, and the large reservoir of asymptomatic female carriers. Of lesser importance is the fact that many strains of *N. gonorrhoeae* are decreasingly sensitive to penicillin.

Probably the most important obstacle in the control of gonorrhea is the asymptomatic female carrier. A high percentage of infected females are completely symptom free and are unaware of their infection. These carriers provide the reservoir that serves to perpetuate the infection within the population. This problem is illustrated by a study carried out in an urban hospital in Brooklyn, New York, where smears and cultures from the urethra, cervix, and anal canal of 875 consecutive patients were examined for gonorrhea. Seventy-two cases of gonorrhea were proved, giving an infection rate of 8.2% [24].

Although *N. gonorrhoeae* is unable to penetrate the skin, penetration and infection of the mucosa occurs readily. In males the urethra is attacked first, resulting in purulent urethritis and involvement of urethral glands. The incubation period varies from two to eight days. There is a sudden onset of dysuria, urgency, and frequency associated with mucoid urethral discharge. Gonococcal urethritis usually does not cause fever, but direct spread of infection may result in prostatitis, epididymitis, or seminal vesiculitis. These infections are frequently associated with fever. Acute urinary retention may result from prostatitis. Gonococcal proctitis in the male is almost always the result of rectal intercourse. Untreated gonorrhea subsides over a period of weeks although gonococci may persist, usually in the prostate. Urethral stricture is a common sequela of untreated urethritis, especially after recurrent attacks. Epididymitis can result in sterility.

In the female, urethritis is mild and transient, although Bartholin's and Skene's glands and glands of the cervix may become infected. Contiguous spread of infection can result in salpingitis or proctitis; ascent of infection to the fallopian tubes usually occurs during or just after menstruation. Gonococcal salpingitis is generally bilateral and may result in a pyosalpinx and formation of tuboovarian abscesses. This tends to heal with fibrosis and adhesions that may produce obstruction and sterility. In females the disease may begin with dysuria, urgency, and frequency after an incubation period of two to eight days. The urethritis is frequently of short duration and often is quite mild. Dissemination of gonococcal infection frequently occurs during menstruation, presumably because the number of organisms shed through the cervix is maximal at this time [25]. The vagina does not usually become infected in adults, probably because of the presence of stratified squamous epithelium with many layers of cells and no glands. Although endometrial infection occurs when gonococci invade the fallopian tubes, it is not serious and subsides promptly.

One of the important reasons for the continuing rise in the incidence of gonorrhea in this country is the difficulty of identifying women with unsuspected or asymptomatic gonorrhea. They not only contribute to the perpetuation of the infection in the population, but they also are candidates for the more destructive later complications of the disease. A number of historical factors have led to the conclusion that many females are asymptomatic carriers of this disease: the ratio of men to women in reported cases is about 8:1, 80% of women known to be infected are asymptomatic, and surveys of female populations, such as those found in obstetric clinics, have indicated that *N. gonorrhoeae* can be cultured in about 5 to 10% of patients. The percentage of positive cultures will vary somewhat with the method used, the number of cultures taken, and the population studied. A recent gonorrhea screening survey by the U.S. Public Health Service indicates that of 143,942 tests, the percentage of positive cultures varied from 32% in venereal disease clinics to 6% in public hospital outpatient clinics, 6% in student health centers, 5% in private hospital outpatient clinics, and to 2% in private clinics [26].

Diagnosis of Gonorrhea

The original technique to demonstrate gonococci, microscopical examination of stained exudates for gram-negative diplococci within polymorphonuclear leukocytes, continues to provide an easy and sensitive method to detect gonococci in men with urethral discharges. In women, however, an examination of smears of cervical or urethral exudates is far too insensitive even in the best of hands and is only used as an adjunct to a cervical culture. In neither sex does a negative smear exclude gonorrhea; cultures should always be performed before nongonococcal urethritis or cervicitis is considered. Likewise, a negative smear is an inadequate test for cure after antibiotic therapy. Occasionally a smear will be positive but no organisms are grown in culture. This is usually due to ineffective culture technique, but the possibility of a false-positive smear should be considered. Garson and Thayer [27] found saprophytic *Neisseria* in 3.4% of women not infected with gonorrhea.

Since direct smears are relatively insensitive and the processing of cultures is sometimes difficult, a cooperative study was undertaken to determine the effectiveness of the fluorescent antibody staining technique [28]. This was an extension of the 1959 study of Deacon and co-workers, who found that successful identification of *N. gonorrhoeae* by fluorescent antibody methods was practical [29]. The nationwide study of Lucas et al. [28] showed that when the fluorescent antibody technique was applied to direct smears of exudates, it lacked the necessary sensitivity. However, when the delayed fluorescent antibody method was used, results improved considerably.

The delayed fluorescent antibody method consists of a direct inoculation of a culture slant with incubation under carbon dioxide, and fluorescent antibody staining of a smear made from the slant. The increase in the number of gonococci during incubation improves the sensitivity and yields results comparable to direct cultures with a substantial saving of time. However, the method depends upon the production of high-titer, specific conjugates, a difficult process which requires careful standardization. In addition, other bacteria may stain with specific antigonococcal antisera unless the antiserum is absorbed with these organisms prior to its use [30]. A disadvantage of this technique is that the delayed fluorescent antibody test is unsatisfactory as a criterion of cure, since gonococci killed by therapy continue to stain. In the experience of Deacon et al. [29], the delayed method of antibody identification was not significantly superior to the conventional culture for the detection of the gonococcus in female contacts of patients with gonorrhea. Its chief advantage was the decreased time necessary to identify the gonococcus—approximately 20 hours as compared with as long as ten days for cultures that required purification measures before definitive identification could be made.

The results of these investigations may be summarized as follows: for the primary diagnosis of gonorrhea in the female, the Thayer-Martin culture and the delayed fluorescent antibody technique are of equal efficiency if multiple sites are examined. However, if examinations are limited to specimens from only one site, culture will be significantly more productive than the delayed method in the examination of specimens from the cervix and especially so in examination of specimens from the vagina.

Techniques of Culture. The major problem in culturing the gonococcus was resolved in 1964 by the development of a sensitive medium for the isolation of the pathogenic *Neisseria* by Thayer and Martin [31]. Improved Thayer-Martin (T-M) medium incorporates vancomycin, colistimethate, and nystatin. This combination of antibiotics reduces the overgrowth by contaminating organisms and improves the specificity of the presumptive identification of *N. gonorrhoeae.* The inhibition of the saprophytic *Neisseria* is nearly complete, and *Mima polymorpha* variant *oxidans,* another organism that might be mistaken for the gonococcus, is also inhibited. Three criteria should be filled to identify an isolated organism as a gonococcus: growth on T-M medium, a positive oxidase reaction, and typical gram-negative diplococcal morphology. Confirmatory tests such as sugar fermentation or fluorescent antibody staining need not be done.

In order to obtain a high yield of positive cultures, fresh medium should be inoculated at the time the patient is examined. The use of transport media and nonselective agar will yield fewer positive cultures. There is a transport medium available, Transgrow (Difco Laboratories, BBL), designed specifically for pathogenic *Neisseria* which appears to be reliable. Nevertheless, direct inoculation of T-M selective medium is the preferred method. In men one should culture all urethral discharges in which a gram stain is not conclusively positive. In women the specific sites available for culture become of definite significance, since the percentages of positive cultures vary with the site used. If one examines a group of asymptomatic female carriers proved by positive culture and determines which locations are most likely to yield a positive result, the following will occur: the cervix will be positive in 94%, the rectum will be positive in 49%, the urethra and vagina will each be positive in about 78%. When these data are recombined in order to show which culture site combination might be used to give the highest yield on a single visit, the following data emerge: cervix and rectum yield 100% positive and cervix and urethra or vagina yield about 94% positive cultures; other combinations yield a significantly lower number of positive cultures [32]. Therefore, when one examines a woman for the presence of asymptomatic gonorrhea, one should culture both the cervix and the anal canal in order to maximize the possibility for a positive cultural result.

The technique for culture is relatively simple: a sterile cotton-tipped applicator is used to swab the endocervix and is immediately rolled onto T-M medium (or chocolate agar if the former is not available) and placed in a candle jar at room temperature. The anal canal is cultured in the same manner, although if fecal material is obtained on the end of the swab it should be discarded and a second swab taken. The cultures should be incubated as soon as possible, since *Neisseria* are relatively thermosensitive and will not grow at temperatures markedly below 37°C.

Treatment of Gonorrhea

Despite the many variations and combinations of antibiotics which have been used for the treatment of gonorrhea, penicillin remains the drug of choice despite the problem of slowly developing resistance of the organism to the drug. During the decade which followed World War II, therapeutic success correlated well with in vitro sensitivity of gonococcal strains [33]. Increasing treatment failure has been paralleled by increasing in vitro antibiotic resistance [34], and the average sensitivity of gonococcal strains obtained from treatment failures has increased from 0.1 units of penicillin per milliliter in 1954 to 0.5 units per milliliter in 1969. The principles of treatment are, however, unchanged. Suboptimal doses of antibiotics should not be used; low blood and tissue levels of antibiotics resulting from inadequate dosage or sustained-release preparations may selectively kill the more sensitive strains and allow the more resistant strains to grow. Thus benzathine penicillin, which is quite effective in the treatment of syphilis, is ineffective in the treatment of gonorrhea. Second, adequate duration of effective in vivo antibiotic activity should be provided. Probenecid may be used in conjunction with a single dose of penicillin or ampicillin to retard urinary secretion and provide higher, more sustained blood levels. Oral preparations of penicillin may not provide adequate blood levels because of variable gastrointestinal absorption. Moreover, many patients are not reliable enough to be expected to complete a full course of oral therapy. There is no evidence to indicate that combinations of antibiotics are of any value in the treatment of gonorrhea. Finally, a test of cure should be routine on all patients; this consists of follow-up cultures obtained about one week after therapy. These follow-up cultures should be obtained from both the cervix and rectum in order to maximize the possibility of a positive result.

The therapeutic recommendations of the U.S. Public Health Service are as follows: aqueous procaine penicillin G, 4.8 million units intramuscularly divided into at least two doses and injected at different sites at one visit, together with 1 gm. of oral probenecid, preferably given at least 30 minutes prior to the injection. This regimen is effective for men or women. An alternative method for oral treatment is the use of ampicillin, 3.5 gm., with probenecid, 1 gm., administered simultaneously. Patients with known exposure to gonorrhea should receive the same treatment as those known to have gonorrhea. Persons with penicillin hypersensitivity or in whom the above regimens have failed to eliminate the disease may be given spectinomycin intramuscularly. The dose for men is 2 gm. and for women, 4 gm. An alternate oral regimen is tetracycline, 1.5 gm. initially followed by 0.5 gm. four times a day for four days; the total dose is 9 gm. Other tetracyclines are no more effective than tetracycline hydrochloride. Erythromycin, 500 mg. every 6 hours for five days, may be substituted during pregnancy.

Follow-up urethral cultures should be obtained from males seven days after completion of treatment; cervical and rectal cultures should be obtained from females at seven to fourteen days after completion of treatment. All patients with gonorrhea should have a serologic test for syphilis at the time of diagnosis. Patients receiving the recommended parenteral penicillin schedule need not have follow-up serologic tests for syphilis. Patients treated with ampicillin, spectinomycin, or tetracycline should have a follow-up serologic test for syphilis each month for four months to detect syphilis that may have been masked by treatment for gonorrhea.

Patients with gonorrhea who also have syphilis should be given additional treatment appropriate to the stage of syphilis.

REFERENCES

1. King, A. Failure to control venereal disease. *Brit. Med. J.* 1:451, 1970.
2. Center for Disease Control. Summaries of reported cases of infectious syphilis. *Morbid. Mortal. Weekly Rep.* 19:360, 1970.
3. Fleming, W. L., Brown, W. J., Donohue, J. F., and Branigin, P. W. National survey of venereal disease treated by physicians in 1968. *J.A.M.A.* 211:1827, 1970.
4. Gjestland, T. The Oslo study of untreated syphilis: An epidemiologic investigation of the natural course of the syphilitic infection based upon a re-study of the Boech-Bruusgaard material. *Acta Dermatovener.* (Stockholm) (Suppl. 34), 1955.
5. World Health Organization. Report of a scientific group on treponematoses research. *W.H.O. Techn. Rep. Ser.* No. 455, 1970.
6. Wallace, A. L., and Norins, L. G. Syphilis Serology Today. In M.

Stefanini (Ed.), *Progress in Clinical Pathology*, Vol. 2. New York: Grune & Stratton, 1969. Pp. 198–215.
7. Dandoy, S. Initial serological reactions in infectious syphilis. *Brit. J. Vener. Dis.* 43:105, 1967.
8. Fiumara, J. J. Biologic false-positive reaction for syphilis: Massachusetts, 1954–1961. *New Eng. J. Med.* 268:402, 1963.
9. Moore, J. E., and Mohr, C. F. Biologically false positive serologic tests for syphilis: Type, incidence and cause. *J.A.M.A.* 150:467, 1952.
10. Cherubin, C. E., and Millian, S. J. Serologic investigations in narcotic addicts: I. Syphilis, lymphogranuloma venereum, herpes simplex, and Q fever. *Ann. Intern. Med.* 69:739, 1968.
11. Carr, R. D., Becker, S. W., and Carpenter, C. M. The biological false-positive phenomenon in elderly men. *Arch. Derm.* (Chicago) 93:393, 1965.
12. Litwin, S. D., and Singer, J. M. Studies of the incidence and significance of anti-gamma globulin factors in the aging. *Arthritis Rheum.* 8:538, 1965.
13. Edmundson, W. F., Ackerman, J. H., Gutierrez-Salinas, E., and Olansky, S. Study of the TPI test in clinical syphilis: 1. Untreated early symptomatic syphilis. *A.M.A. Arch. Derm. Syph.* 70:298, 1954.
14. Deacon, W. E., and Hunter, E. F. Treponemal antigens as related to identification and syphilis serology. *Proc. Soc. Exp. Biol. Med.* 110:352, 1962.
15. Sever, J. L. Immunoglobulin determinations for the detection of perinatal infections. *J. Pediat.* 75:1111, 1969.
16. Alford, C. A., Schaefer, J., Blankenship, W. J., Straumfjord, J. V., and Cassady, G. E. A correlative immunologic microbiologic and clinical approach to the diagnosis of acute and chronic infections in newborn infants. *New Eng. J. Med.* 277:437, 1967.
17. Alford, C. A., Jr., Polt, S. S., Cassady, G. E., Straumfjord, J. V., and Remington, J. S. γM-fluorescent treponemal antibody in the diagnosis of congenital syphilis. *New Eng. J. Med.* 280:1086, 1969.
18. Syphilis: a Synopsis. (U.S. Public Health Service Publication No. 1660). Washington, D.C.: Government Printing Office, 1968.
19. Lucas, J. B., and Price, E. V. Co-operative evaluation of treatment for early syphilis: Preliminary report with special reference to spectinomycin sulphate (actinospectacin). *Brit. J. Vener. Dis.* 43:244–248, 1967.
20. Collart, P., Borel, L-J., and Durel, P. Significance of spiral organisms found, after treatment, in late human and experimental syphilis. *Brit. J. Vener. Dis.* 40:81, 1964.
21. Smith, J. L., and Israel, C. W. The presence of spirochetes in late seronegative syphilis. *J.A.M.A.* 199:980, 1967.
22. Smith, J. L., and Israel, C. W. Treponemes in aqueous humor in late seronegative syphilis. *Trans. Amer. Acad. Opthal. Otolaryng.* 72:63, 1968.
23. Montenegro, E. N. R., Nicol, W. G., and Smith, J. L. Treponemalike forms and artifacts. *Amer. J. Opthal.* 68:197, 1969.
24. Cave, V. G., Bloomfield, R. D., Hurdle, E. S., Gordon, E. W., Hammock, D. Gonorrhea in the obstetric and gynecologic clinic. *J.A.M.A.* 210:309, 1969.

25. Holmes, K. K., Counts, G. W., and Beaty, H. N. Disseminated gonococcal infection. *Ann. Intern. Med.* 74:979, 1971.
26. Schroeter, A. L., and Pazin, G. T. Gonorrhea. *Ann. Intern. Med.* 72:553, 1970.
27. Thayer, J. D., and Garson, W. The Gonococcus. In R. J. Dubos and J. G. Hirsch (Eds.), *Bacterial and Mycotic Infections of Man* (4th ed.). Philadelphia: Lippincott, 1965. P. 451.
28. Lucas, J. B., Price, E. V., Thayer, J. D., and Schroeter, A. L. Diagnosis and treatment of gonorrhea in the female. *New Eng. J. Med.* 276:1454, 1967.
29. Deacon, W. E., et al. Identification of *Neisseria gonorrhea* by means of fluorescent antibodies. *Proc. Soc. Exp. Biol. Med.* 101:322, 1959.
30. Lind, I. Identification of *Neisseria gonorrhoeae* by means of fluorescent antibody technique. *Acta Path. Microbiol. Scand.* 70:613, 1967.
31. Thayer, J. D., and Martin, J. E. Improved medium selective for cultivation of *N. gonorrhoeae* and *N. meningitidis. Public Health Rep.* 81:569, 1966.
32. Schmale, J. D., Martin, J. E., and Domescik, G. Observations on the culture diagnosis of gonorrhea in women. *J.A.M.A.* 210:312, 1969.
33. Guthe, T. Failure to control gonorrhea. *Bull. W.H.O.* 24:297, 1961.
34. Martin, J. E., Lester, A., Price, E. U., et al. Comparative Study of Gonococcal Susceptibility to Penicillin in Metropolitan Areas of the United States. Presented at Ninth Interscience Conference on Antimicrobial Agents and Chemotherapy, Oct. 27, 1969, Washington, D.C.
35. Deacon, W. E., Lucas, J. B., and Price, E. U. Fluorescent treponemal antibody-absorption (FTA-ABS) test for syphilis. *J.A.M.A.* 198:624, 1966.
36. Sparling, P. F. Diagnosis and treatment of syphilis. *New Eng. J. Med.* 284:642, 1971.

INDEX

Achromobacter organisms, 39, 64
Acquired valvular disease, 100
Actinomyces and nocardia, 45–46
Actinomyces israeli, 46, 138
Adenosine arabinoside, 138
Adenoviruses, 48–49
Alcaligenes organisms, 39
Allergic bronchopulmonary disorders, 47
Amantidine, 48
Aminoglycosides, 83
  mechanism of action, 5
  in renal failure, 26–27
Amphotericin B, 21, 138
Ampicillin, 8, 46
  gram-negative septicemia, 93
  in renal failure, 22, 23, 28
Anaerobes, 42–43
Antibiotic therapy, 17. *See also under specific name*
  bacterial endocarditis, 107–108
    prophylactic antibiotics, 109–110
  dosage, 5
  gonorrhea, 168–169
  macrolide, 7, 12–14
  oral administration, 4–5
  parenteral route, 5
  reasons for ineffectiveness of treatment, 6
  in renal failure, 5–6, 17–29
    general guidelines, 21–28
  sensitivity determinations, 2–3, 6
  streptococcal disease, 151
  therapeutic decisions, 5
Antibody deficiency, 131–132
Antimicrobial agents, 1
  identification of etiologic agent, 1
  mechanism of action, 4–5
  therapeutic alternatives to penicillin, 7–16
Arthritis, 145
Aspergillosis, 134
Azotemia, 106
  antibiotics in renal failure, 22

Bacitracin, mechanism of action, 5
Bacteremia, 88, 90
Bacterial endocarditis, 97–111
  acute, 98
  bacteriology, 102–103
  complication of hemodialysis, 101–102
  diagnosis, 103–106
    cardiac manifestations, 104–105

Bacterial endocarditis, diagnosis—*Continued*
embolic phenomena, 105
hypersensitivity reactions, 105
metastatic infection, 104
neurological manifestations, 105
nonspecific symptoms, 104
renal lesions, 106
rheumatoid factor, 105–106
following open-heart surgery, 100
intravenous drug use, 101
laboratory tests, 3–4, 106
pathogenesis, 98–102
acquired valvular disease, 100
congenital heart disease, 99–100
underlying disease, 99–100
subacute, 3, 98
treatment, 106–110
assessment of, 109
enterococci, 108
gram-negative bacteria, 108
with negative cultures, 108
penicillin-sensitive patients, 108–109
principles of therapy, 106–107
prophylactic therapy, 109–110
relapse after, 109
specific pathogens, 107–108
Staphylococcus aureus or *epidermidis,* 107–108
surgery, 108
Bacterial meningitis. *See* Meningitis, bacterial
Bactericidal agents, 4–5
mechanisms of action, 4–5
Bacteriostatic agents, 4–5
mechanisms of action, 5
Bacteriuria, 76–77. *See also* Urinary tract infections
asymptomatic, 78–80
chronic, 80–82
modes of therapy, 81
Bacteroides, 42–43, 133, 138
septicemia, 93–94
Bagassosis, 47
Biliary tract infection, 5–6. *See also* Renal failure
Bones (osteomyelitis), etiologic agents, 3
Bronchial brush biopsy, 33
Bronchiolitis, 41, 48, 49
Bronchitis, 41
erythromycin therapy, 13
Bronchopneumonia, 40, 41
Bronchoscopy, 33

Candida infections, 3, 101, 133, 137, 138
Carbenicillin, 8
gram-negative septicemia, 93
in renal failure, 23
urinary tract infections, 82
Cellular immunity, 131
Cephalexin, 11–12
in renal failure, 22, 24, 28
dose-level modifications, 23
toxic reaction, 11–12
urinary tract infections, 83
Cephaloridine, 11
avoided in renal failure, 21, 22, 27
Cephalosporins, 10–12
mechanisms of action, 5
in renal failure, 21, 22
dose-interval modifications, 23
Cephalothin, 11
in renal failure, 23, 24
Chemotherapeutic agents, 21–28. *See also* Antibiotic therapy
avoided in renal insufficiency, 27–28
dose-interval modifications
agents of low toxicity, 23
agents with significant toxicity, 25
tuberculosis patients, 121
excreted by both renal and nonrenal mechanisms, 22–24
excreted primarily by renal mechanisms, 24–27
for urinary tract infections with uremia, 28
Children and infants
neonatal meningitis, 53–56
respiratory tract infections, 41–42
urinary tract infections, 74, 76, 83
Chlamydiae, pulmonary infections, 43
Chloramphenicol, 4, 43, 45, 69
gram-negative septicemia, 93
mechanism of action, 5
in renal failure, 21, 24
Chloroquine, in renal failure, 21
Chlortetracycline, in renal failure, 21
Clindamycin, 14, 43

Cloxacillin, 9–10
Coliform organism, 132–133
Colistimethate, in renal failure, 25
Colistin (polymyxin E), 69
Concentration of drugs in serum, 17–18
Conjunctivitis, inclusion, 43
Contamination, 125–126
  covering nose and mouth, 125
  ultraviolet light, 126
  ventilation and, 125–126
Coryza (common cold), 48, 49
Coxicella burnetii, 44
Creatine clearance, 19–21
Croup, 48, 49
Cultures, 2
  general rules, 2
  gonorrhea, 167–168
  opportunistic infections, 136–137
  pour plates, 2
  sputum, 2, 32
  surgical and postmortem lung, 31
Cytomegalovirus, 48–49, 134, 138
Cytosine arabinoside, 48, 138

Dermatophytes, 3
Dicloxacillin, 9
Diplococcus pneumoniae, 3, 34–36, 64, 98
Drug addiction and bacterial endocarditis, 101
Drugs, 4–5, 17–21
  absorption, 17
  bactericidal, 4–5
  bacteriostatic, 4–5
  concentration in serum, 17–18
  creatine clearance, 19–21
  distribution, 17
  excretion of, 18–19
  measurement of serum drug levels, 17–18
  metabolism, 17

Ear infections, etiologic agents, 3
Eczema vaccinatum, 135
Encephalitis, 63
Endocarditis, bacterial. *See* Bacterial endocarditis
Endotoxin, systemic effects in central nervous system meningitis, 59–62
Enterobacter, 38, 64, 93
Enterococci, 38, 103, 108, 146
Epidemiology, streptococcal infections, 149–150
Epiglottitis, acute, 41
Erythromycin, 12–13, 69
  mechanism of action, 5
  in renal failure, 21, 24
Escherichia coli, 3, 8, 55, 59, 64, 78, 81, 87, 90, 93
Ethambutol, for treating tuberculosis, 121, 122
Etiologic agents, 1–3
  identification of, 1–2
  more common infections, 2–3

Farmer's lung, 47
Fungi
  opportunistic infections, 46–47, 133–134
  pulmonary infections, 46–47
  therapy for infections, 138
  yeastlike, 133

Gentamicin
  gram-negative septicemia, 93
  in renal failure, 25, 27
  urinary tract infections, 82–83
Glomerulonephritis, strep infection, 143, 150, 151, 159
Gonorrhea, 164–169
  diagnosis of, 165–168
    cervical cultures, 166
    delayed fluorescent antibody method, 166–167
    microscopic examination, 165–166
    techniques of culture, 167–168
  in females, 165
  incidence of, 164
  in males, 164
  obstacles to control, 164–165
  transmission, 164
  treatment, 168–169
Gram-negative bacteria, 2, 38–43, 90
  bacterial endocarditis, 108
  meningitis, 68–69
Gram-negative bacteremia, 88
Gram-negative septicemia, 87–95
  antibiotic therapy, 93–94
  bacteriology, 90
  incidence of, 87
  pathophysiology, 88–90

Gram-negative septicemia—*Continued*
predisposing conditions, 90–91
prevention, 95
prognosis, 94–95
treatment, 91–94
antibiotic therapy, 93–94
therapy of shock, 91–93
Gram-positive bacteria, 2, 34–38
penicillin G for treating, 7
therapeutic alternatives to penicillin, 7–16
Gram stain, 2
common errors in using, 2
culturing and, 2

Haemophilus influenzae, 3, 36, 41–42, 56, 64
ampicillin for, 8
meningitis, 66–68
Hageman factor (XII), 89
Hemodialysis, endocarditis as complication of, 101–102
Hepatitis, 134
Herellea organism, 39
Herpes simplex, 108, 134
Herpes viruses, 49, 137
Herpes zoster, 132, 134
Hodgkin's disease, 135
Hospitals
treatment of tuberculosis, 124–126
urinary tract infections, 83–84
Host defense mechanisms, 1, 5
general considerations, 5
opportunistic infections, 129–132
Hypersensitivity reactions, bacterial endocarditis, 105

Immune deficiency, 131–132
Immunity
cellular, 131
syphilis, 157–159
Infectious mononucleosis, 49
Infective endovasculitis, 97. *See also* Bacterial endocarditis
Influenza, 48–49
Haemophilus influenzae, 3, 36, 41–42, 56, 64
ampicillin for, 8
meningitis, 66–68
INH. *See* Isoniazid
Inhalation therapy and pulmonary infections, 39–40
Intravenous drugs, administration of, 4
Iodode oxyuridine, 138
Isoniazid, 119–121
associated liver disease, 21, 119–120
preventive therapy, 120–121
in renal failure, 21, 119–120
Isoxazolyl penicillins, 9, 10

Joints, microorganisms commonly isolated from, 3

Kanamycin, 93
in renal failure, 25, 27
Kidney diseases, guidelines for drug administration, 17. *See also* Renal failure
Kinin system, 89
Klebsiella organisms, 8, 11
gram-negative bacteria, 38–39, 93–94
Klebsiella pneumoniae, 36, 38
Klebsiella-Aerobacter species, 78
Klebsiella-Enterobacter, 55, 90, 133

Laboratory tests, 2
antibiotic discs, 3
bacterial endocarditis, 116
bacterial meningitis, 63
general considerations, 2
gram stain, 2
pulmonary infections, 31–34
streptococci, 146–148
Laryngitis, 48, 49
Leukemia, 132
Lincomycin, 7, 13–14
derivatives, 12–14
mechanism of action, 5
in renal failure, 21, 24
Liver diseases, guidelines for drug administration, 17
Lung infections
etiologic agents, 3
farmer's lung, 47
surgical lung cultures, 34
Lymphogranuloma venereum, 43
Lymphoma, 21
Lysosomal enzymes, 89

Macrolide antibiotics, 7, 12–14
Maple bark disease, 47
Measles (rubeola), 48–49
Melioidosis, 40

Meningitis, bacterial, 53–69
in children and adults, 56–57
diagnosis, 62–63
effects of endotoxin in central nervous system, 59–62
etiology, 64–69
gram-negative organisms, 68–69
Haemophilus influenzae, 66–68
meningococcus meningitis, 65–66
staphylococcus, 68
laboratory tests, 63
neonatal, 53–56, 145
pathogenesis and prognosis, 57–59
pneumococcal, 57–58
symptoms, 56–57
therapy, 64–69
in persons allergic to penicillin, 69
Methenamine mandelate (Mandelamine), 82
avoided in renal failure, 27
Methicillin, 8–9, 10
in renal failure, 23
Microcirculation, 89
Microorganisms, isolated from acute adult infections, 3
Mima organisms, 39, 167
Mycobacterium kansasii, 114, 116, 118
Mycobacterium tuberculosis, 114, 115, 118
Mycoplasma, pulmonary infections, 43–44
Mycoplasma hominis, 43
Mycoplasma pneumoniae, 3, 13, 43

Nafcillin, 9–10
Nalidixic acid, mechanism of action, 5
Neisseria gonorrhoeae, 3, 164, 167
Neisseria meningitidis, 3, 64, 65
Nephrotic syndrome, 132
Nitrofurantoin, 5
avoided in renal failure, 27, 28
urinary tract infections, 79
Nocardia asteroides, 138
Nocardiosis, 45–46

Oleandomycin, 12
Opportunistic bacilli, gram-negative, 39–41
Opportunistic infections, 129–142
diagnosis, 136–138
etiologic agents, 132–136
bacteria, 132–133
fungi, 133–134
protozoa, 135–136
viruses, 134–135
fungi and, 46–47, 133–134
host defenses, 129–132
therapy, 138–139
preventive, 139
Oral therapy, 4–5
Osteomyelitis, etiologic agents, 3
Oxacillin, 9–10
in renal failure, 23

Para-aminosalicylic acid (PASA)
avoided in renal failure, 27–28
for tuberculosis, 122
Paracolobactrum, 55
Parainfluenza, 48–49
Parasitic infections, 47–48
PASA. *See* Para-aminosalicylic acid
Penicillin G, 7–8, 46
in renal failure, 22, 23
Penicillin V, 8
Penicillins, 4–5, 7–16
allergic reactions
therapy for bacterial endocarditis, 108–109
therapy for meningitis, 69
cephalosporins, 10–12
cephalexin, 11–12
cephaloridine, 11
cephalothin, 11
dose-level modifications, 23
for gonorrhea, 168–169
lincomycin derivatives, 12–14
macrolide antibiotics, 12–14
mechanism of action, 4–5
in renal failure, 21, 22
dose-interval modifications, 23
semisynthetic, 7–10
carbenicillin, 8
isoxazolyl penicillins, 9–10
methicillin, 8–10
penicillin G, 7–8, 22, 46
streptococcal disease, 151–152
urinary tract infections, 79
vancomycin, 14–15
Percutaneous transthoracic aspiration, 33
Peritonitis, pneumococcal, 132
Phagocytosis, 130–131

Pharyngitis, 43–44, 48, 49
  streptococcal infection, 145, 149–150
Phycomycosis, 134
Pleurodynia, 48–49
Pneumococcal lobar pneumonia, 34–36
Pneumocystis carinii, 47, 135–137
Pneumonia
  Diplococcus pneumoniae, 3, 34–36, 64, 98
  erythromycin therapy, 13
  gram-positive bacteria, 34–36
  interstitial, 47–48
  Klebsiella, 38–39
  lobar, 34–36
  mycoplasma, 3, 13, 43–44
  necrotizing, 40
  P. carinii, 135–137
  staphylococcal, 37–38
  streptococcal, 36
  viruses, 48–49
Polymyxins, 5, 69
  gram-negative septicemia, 93
  mechanism of action, 5
  in renal failure, 27
Pregnancy
  bacteriuria during, 74, 76–77
  urinary tract infections, 74, 76–77
Proteus mirabilis, 8
Proteus species, 8, 38, 55, 78, 82, 90, 93–94, 133
Protozoa, opportunistic infections, 135–136
Pseudomonas aeruginosa, 8, 40, 82, 90, 130
Pseudomonas organisms, 11, 39, 55, 68, 78–79, 90, 93–94, 101, 132
Pseudomonas pseudomallei, 41
Psittacosis, 43
Pulmonary infections, 31–52
  actinomyces and nocardia, 45–46
  chlamydiae, 43
  diagnostic procedures, 31–34
    bronchial brush biopsy, 33
    bronchoscopy, 33
    percutaneous transthoracic aspiration, 33–34
    sputum culture, 32
    sputum smear, 32
    surgical and postmortem lung cultures, 34
    transtracheal aspiration, 32–33
  etiologic categories, 34–38
  fungi, 46–47
  gram-negative bacteria, 38–43
    Bacteroides and related anaerobes, 42–43
    Enterobacteriaceae, 38
    Klebsiellae, 38–39
    opportunistic bacilli, 39–41
  gram-positive bacteria, 34–36
    Diplococcus pneumoniae, 34–36
    enterococcus, 38
    Staphylococcus aureus, 36–38
    Staphylococcus epidermidis, 37
    Streptococcus pyogenes, 36
  mycoplasma, 43–44
  parasitic infections, 47–48
  rickettsiae, 44–45
  viruses, 48–49
Pyelonephritis, 76–77
  acute, 80
Pyoderma, 150
Pyrazinamide (PZA) for treating tuberculosis, 121–123

Q fever, 44–45

Reflux, vesicoureteral, 83
Renal failure
  agents excreted by both renal and nonrenal mechanisms, 22–24
  agents excreted primarily by renal mechanisms, 24–27
  agents to be avoided, 27–28
  antibiotic regimes, 6, 17–29
    general guidelines, 21–28
  drugs for tuberculosis and, 121
  treatment of urinary tract infections in uremia, 28
Renal lesions, bacterial endocarditis, 106
Respiratory syncytial virus, 49
Respiratory syndromes, 48
Rheumatic fever
  acute, 150–152
  streptococci, 143, 145, 150, 151
Rheumatoid factor, bacterial endocarditis, 105–106
Rickettsiae, 44–45
Rifampicin, 5
  for treating tuberculosis, 123

Salmonella species, 3, 8, 38, 55, 132, 133
Scarlet fever, 148–150
Sensitivity testing of organisms, 2–3
Septicemia, 133
  gram-negative. *See* Gram-negative septicemia
Sequoiosis, 47
Serologic tests
  opportunistic infections, 137
  syphilis, 159–162
Serratia, 38
Serum drug levels, measurement of, 17
Shigella species, 8, 35, 59
Shock, gram-negative septicemia, 91–93
Sickle cell disease, 132
Sinuses, paranasal infections, 3
Skin and subcutaneous tissue infections, 3
Smallpox vaccination, complications of, 135–136
Sputum, culture and smear, 32
Staphylococcal enterocolitis, 15
Staphylococcus aureus, 3, 36–38, 98, 102, 107–108
Staphylococcus epidermidis, 37, 100, 102, 107–108
Staphylococcus meningitis, 68
Streptococcal disease, 36, 143–153
  attack rates, 143, 150
  epidemiology, 149–150
  immunity, 149–150
  organism, host and clinical syndromes, 148–149
  streptococci, 143–146
    aerobic, 144, 146
    anaerobic, 146
    antigen properties, 144
    classification of, 144
    enterococci, 146
    isolation and identification, 146–148
    methicillin-resistant, 15
    morphology and colonies, 143–144
    viridans, 145–146
  treatment and prophylaxis, 151–152
Streptococcus agalactiae, 145
Streptococcus faecalis, 3
Streptococcus pyogenes, 3, 36
Streptomycin
  in renal failure, 25–27
  in tuberculosis, 121–122
Sulfonamides
  mechanism of action, 5
  in renal failure, 28
  urinary tract infections, 78–79
Syphilis, 155–164
  congenital, 161–162
  immunology, 157–159
    antibodies, 157–158
    cell-mediated immunity, 158
  incidence, 155–156
  nontreponemal tests, 157–159
  serological tests, 159–162
    congenital syphilis, 161–162
    false-positive reactions, 159–160
    fluorescent treponemal antibody, 160–161
    Kolmer, 159
    reactivity at various clinical stages, 161
    treponemal immobilization tests, 160–161
    Venereal Disease Research Laboratory (VDRL) slide tests, 159, 161
  systemic disease, 156
  transmission, 155–156
  treatment, 162–164
    penicillin, 162–164
    persisting treponemas after treatment, 163–164
    U.S. Public Health Service recommendations, 162

Taxoplasma gondii, 135, 137
Taxoplasma infection, 135, 137–138
Tetracyclines, 5, 42, 44, 45
  in renal failure, 25, 26
Therapy, 1–5
  associated diseases and, 5
  general considerations, 1–4
Tonsillitis, 149
Tracheobronchitis, 48, 49
Trachoma, 43
Transtracheal aspiration, 32–33
Treponema pallidum, 155–156, 160, 163
  immobilization test, 160–161
Triacetyloleandomycin, 12

Tricuspid endocarditis, 101
Tuberculosis, 113–127
  in adolescents, 115
  chemotherapy, 118–124
  clinical studies, 114–116
  communicability, 114–115
  drug resistance, 118–119
  ethambutol, 122
  hospital treatment, 124–126
    elimination of contamination, 124–126
    ultraviolet light, 125
  incidence, 113
  isoniazid for treating, 119–121
    associated liver diseases, 21, 119–120
    preventive therapy, 120–121
  management, 117–124
    for advanced, 118
    minimal lesions, 117–118
    moderately advanced, 118
    in renal failure, 121
    triple regimen, 118–119, 124
  Mycobacterium kansasii, 114, 116, 118
  Mycobacterium tuberculosis, 114, 115, 118
  para-aminosalicylic acid, 122
  pathogenesis, 114
  present status, 113
  preventive therapy, 120–121
  pyrazinamide (PZA), 122–123
  rifampicin, 123
  skin-test reactivity, 113, 115–116
  streptomycin therapy, 121–122

Ulcers, decubitus, 3
Ultraviolet light, for preventing contamination, 126
Uremia
  antibiotics in renal failure, 17
    dose-interval modifications, 22–23
  treatment of urinary tract infections, 28
Urinary tract infections, 73–84
  children and infants, 74, 76, 83
  demonstration of significant bacteriuria, 77–78
  enterococci, 146
  etiologic agents, 3
  incidence, 73–74
  lower tract, 78
  pregnant women, 74, 76–77
  prevention of hospital-acquired, 83–84
  recurrence of, 73–76
  renal involvement, 73
  therapy, 78–83
    antimicrobial agents, newer, 82–83
    asymptomatic bacteriuria, 78–80
    carbenicillin, 82
    cephalexin, 83
    chronic recurrent, 80–82
    gentamicin, 82–83
    upper urinary tract, 78, 80
    in uremia, 28
  vesicoureteral reflux, 83
  in women, 73–74, 76

Vaccinia, 134–135
  eczema vaccinatum, 135
Vaccinia gangrenosa, 135
Vancomycin, 7, 14–15
  mechanism of action, 5
  in renal failure, 25, 27–28
Varicella-zoster infections, 48–49, 138
Venereal disease, 155–171. *See also* Gonorrhea; Syphilis
  epidemiology, 155
  gonorrhea, 164–169
  incidence, 155–156, 164–165
  syphilis, 155–164
Ventilation and contamination, 125–126
Vesicoureteral reflux, 83
Viridans streptococci, 145–146
Viruses
  eczema vaccinatum, 135
  generalized vaccinia, 134–135
  opportunistic infections, 134–135
  respiratory syndromes, 48–49
  therapy, 138
  vaccinia gangrenosa, 135